Health Communication

D1598756

Health Communication

Theoretical and Critical Perspectives

Ruth Cross, Sam Davis
and Ivy O'Neil

polity

First published in 2017 by Polity Press

Polity Press
65 Bridge Street
Cambridge CB2 1UR, UK

Polity Press
350 Main Street
Malden, MA 02148, USA

ISBN-13: 978-0-7456-9772-7 (hardback)
ISBN-13: 978-0-7456-9773-4 (paperback)

A catalogue record for this book is available from the British Library.

Library of Congress Cataloging-in-Publication Data

Names: Cross, Ruth, author. | Davis, Sam, 1968- author. | O'Neil, Ivy, author.
Title: Health communication : theoretical and critical perspectives / Ruth Cross, Sam Davis, Ivy O'Neil.
Description: Cambridge, UK ; Malden, MA : Polity Press, 2017. | Includes bibliographical references and index.
Identifiers: LCCN 2016038602 (print) | LCCN 2016039688 (ebook) | ISBN 9780745697727 (hardback) | ISBN 9780745697734 (pbk.) | ISBN 9780745697758 (Mobi) | ISBN 9780745697765 (Epub)
Subjects: | MESH: Health Communication | Health Behavior | Health Education | Health Promotion | Social Marketing
Classification: LCC RA427.8 (print) | LCC RA427.8 (ebook) | NLM WA 590 | DDC 362.1--dc23
LC record available at https://lccn.loc.gov/2016038602

Typeset in 10.5 on 12 pt Plantin by Servis Filmsetting Ltd, Stockport, Cheshire
Printed and bound in the UK by CPI Group (UK) Ltd, Croydon

For further information on Polity, visit our website: www.politybooks.com

Contents

Detailed Contents

Part II Key Topics

Part III   Issues and Challenges

Acknowledgements

First and foremost we would like to acknowledge the by-proxy contribution that the students we work with have made to this book. Working with them on the Health Communication module in the post-graduate courses that we teach has led to the creation of this work. We appreciate the challenge and fresh insights that our students bring to our academic work as reflected in the debates within this book.

We deeply appreciate the contribution of the reviewers during the process of writing this book. Their helpful and constructive feedback has led to a better final product.

We would like to acknowledge the significant support that we have received from our editorial team at Polity, particularly Jonathan Skerrett, who has kept us on track!

Last, but not least, we must recognize our 'silent' partners in the writing process. Those that have journeyed with us, missed us while we write, listened while we've moaned, brought us copious cups of tea and generally been there over the many months it has taken for us to get from start to finish. A big thank you to our families, our friends and our health promotion colleagues. It would have been much harder without you.

Part I

Theoretical Perspectives

1

Introduction to Health Communication: Theoretical and Critical Perspectives

In this introductory chapter we set the scene for *Health Communication: Theoretical and Critical Perspectives.* We begin by explaining how this book came about and locate health communication within the broader notion of health promotion. We introduce the style of the book and outline the indicative content providing a rationale for the inclusion of the subject matter and emphasizing the global and international outlook of the book. This chapter introduces the three key disciplinary areas which underpin the book's approach – communication, education and psychology. These disciplinary areas link to later chapters and thread through the discussion and debate therein. We also outline the key themes that run through the book in keeping with the ideological, political and philosophical perspectives that underpin it.

This book came about because we, as lecturers of health communication, noted a dearth of more critical perspectives written for a post-graduate and practitioner audience. There are a number of very good undergraduate and practically focused books on health communication on the market which have made a significant contribution to the field. We were conscious, however, that a more in-depth critique of the issues is relatively lacking. Indeed, we have been unable to find a text which focuses solely on health communication with an in-depth insight into the underpinning disciplines and ideology of health promotion and the more critical, analytical research-informed debates on health communication pertinent to post-graduate level. Spotting this gap in the literature we have set out to produce a text which lays bare some of the more sticky issues in health communication as we see them. We unapologetically dismantle what we view as some problematical underpinning assumptions in the field of health communication and turn to a range of critical perspectives to do this. At the outset, however, it is important that we outline our ideological, political and philosophical position since it is against this background that the book is cast.

We teach health communication on the suite of health promotion and public health masters programmes delivered by Leeds Beckett University. Our main discipline, however, is *health promotion* and we subscribe to the values and principles of this discipline. As such the ideological, political and philosophical basis of health promotion sets the context to this book. It is via a 'health promotion' lens that we will view health communication. We adhere to the position that health promotion is the 'militant wing' and 'critical conscience of public health' (Green et al., 2015: 48). What we hope to do in this book is explain this position with regard to health communication. As such, while we do offer insights for reflective practice and suggest implications for practice throughout, we have not written a 'how to do it' text. As previously stated, there are already plenty of good examples of such texts on the market which we would urge readers to turn to if that is what they are looking for. Instead, we have produced a higher level critical textbook on health communication which challenges many of the 'taken for granted', underpinning assumptions of current understanding and practice. We turn to key theoretical and critical perspectives to tease out what we see as the major ideological and political concerns. The book is structured to enable this to take place in a coherent and logical way which, we hope, will aid readers who are relatively new to the debates at hand.

The main purpose of this book is to critically reflect on the assumptions, ideologies and values underpinning well-rehearsed approaches in health communication and, as such, it is aimed at the more advanced reader. This book will appraise health communication and its role in promoting health. Drawing on the evidence base for effectiveness and published international research within the field the book critically considers what works and what does not work in communication for health and health promotion, unpicking common approaches. Moreover, it seeks to scrutinize what we do and why. Crucially the book links theory to practice examining how research relates to real life and what this means for public health and health promotion in our social world.

There is a general assumption that an increase in knowledge directly translates into a change of healthy lifestyle behaviour. The focus of many writers and practitioners is often on why the recipients of health communication efforts do not act on the information and advice given. Increasingly we look to aspects such as message design, health literacy skills, information technologies and social marketing strategies as a means of promoting effectiveness. Recent developments in the use of information communication technology, both software and hardware in health promotion such as internet, social media, mobile devices run through the book and the content is drawn from international research, knowledge and expertise offering a global perspective on the issues raised. In addition we make use of the valuable international health promotion teaching experience we have acquired through working with students on Leeds Beckett courses run in West and sub-Saharan Africa as well as with students who come from all over the world to study on our UK course. We acknowledge the contribution that each of them brings to our growing understanding and appreciation of health communication in a range of contexts.

The ideological, political and philosophical position of health communication: theoretical and critical perspectives

As we briefly outlined earlier, the foundations of this book are located within our ideological, political and philosophical position which mirrors health promotion's disciplinary perspective. Health promotion adheres to a specific set of values and principles which distinguishes it from the broader field of public health. These include empowerment, equity, tackling health inequalities, addressing the social determinants of health, privileging a social model of health, advocacy, ethical practice, participation, collaboration and upstream approaches. As defined by Dixey et al. (2013: 1) we understand health promotion to be 'a social movement with the central aim of tackling the social determinants of health and so bringing about greater social and health justice'. At the outset it is also important to define what we understand by health education as opposed to health promotion. We see health education as an integral part of health promotion but health promotion does not stop there; it goes much further. While health education focuses on the behavioural determinants of health and seeks to address these through preventive and educational efforts aimed largely at the individual, health promotion addresses structural, social and environmental determinants of health as well (Green et al., 2015). So, where does health communication sit within this? We would argue that contemporary health communication practice is more akin to health education than health promotion with its attendant focus on the individual and behaviour change. We aim, in this book, to explain this in some detail. What we would advocate, then, is that health communication adopts approaches which are more ideologically, politically and philosophically akin to health promotion. For example, we privilege the concept of empowerment recognizing the centrality of power in health in all domains. Health communication efforts should, in our opinion, challenge uneven power distribution and advocate for those who are relatively disempowered the challenging of structures, policies and practices which result in subordination and oppression. Therefore the ideological basis of this book is in keeping with the more radical roots of health promotion and this is reflected in the key themes within it that we return to throughout. We will now outline these key themes.

Key themes within health communication: theoretical and critical perspectives

Several important central concepts thread through this book and we will return to them again and again with regard to the different debates. Empowerment is a key concept in health promotion. While open to some debate around definition, conceptualization and measurement empowerment is absolutely central to health promotion (Woodall et al., 2012; Christens, 2013). We advocate empowering approaches in health communication. Linked to this we reject, and are critical of, victim-blaming approaches. Too often health communication efforts result in pointing the finger of blame at individuals or groups who 'fail' to take up advice and change their behaviour without taking into consideration the wider, complex contexts of everyday life. Health promotion takes into account the social, political and environmental factors that influence behavioural choices and practices acknowledging the fundamental importance of these in determining health outcomes. In this book we therefore explore the wider social determinants of health and the influence of these on health communication.

Health promotion is not about telling people what to do or doing things to people, it is about working *with* people. Key to this is true participation. Our position is that health communication efforts should involve the people for whom they are intended. Individuals and communities should be meaningfully engaged in interventions designed to address their concerns. We are therefore critical of top-down, paternalistic and tokenistic means of health communication.

Equity is a key principle of health promotion (Green et al., 2015). Equity is linked to equality. Health promotion is concerned with tackling health inequalities and addressing the gap between the least well-off and most well-off in society. We return to issues of equity and equality throughout the book. Health promotion is predicated on a social model of health which privileges lay perspectives. Health communication efforts often fail because there is a significant disconnect between what the 'experts' say and how this is received and understood by people in the context of their experience (Dutta, 2008). This disconnect can occur for a number of reasons. Often a reductionist, deficit model is used to explain this, the assumption being that people do not understand, misunderstand, cannot make sense of information or are simply irrational (Tulloch and Lupton, 2003; Wilkinson, 2001; Willig, 2008). We consider this to be highly problematic and we are critical of cognition as equated with higher order function. We therefore adopt a non-deficit, non-deviant approach characterized more by an 'assets' model (Morgan and Ziglio, 2007). Rather than focusing on what is problematic, deficient or 'missing' in people asset-based approaches seek to explore, utilize and build upon existing resources, capacities and talents.

We are highly critical of the neoliberal agenda which we see as driving much contemporary health communication practice. Neoliberal discourse creates and emphasizes individual responsibility for health minimizing the role of the state. Neoliberalism is a specific political and economic ideology based on an individualization thesis which emphasizes personal freedom, control and choice which are constructed as freely available to the neoliberal subject (Stuart and Donaghue, 2012). It positions people as autonomous agents directing their own destiny (Rose et al., 2006) and possessing the freedom to transform and reinvent themselves (McRobbie, 2009). Neoliberal ideology has become firmly embedded within so-called 'Western' contexts within the past two decades and now permeates all areas of human experience. The gradual withdrawal of state welfare provision has redirected responsibility to the individual subject (Gill and Scharff, 2011) within the private domain (Bell et al., 2011). In relation to health communication, processes of individualization are reinforced by Western political ideologies which emphasize responsibility and self-determination. The creation of the post-modern, neoliberal subject is reductionist and brings about a problematic lack of attention to the wider determinants of health undermining a progressive agenda. The neoliberal critique is therefore a key theme in this book.

What this book adds to the health communication literature

This book brings communication, education and psychological theories together within one key text. It specifically sets out to challenge assumptions and practice in health communication rather than reiterating well-rehearsed ideas and concepts. It examines the theoretical underpinning of these three disciplines in empowering and motivating change through health communication. This book has greater analytical and critical depth more appropriate to a post-graduate and a critically reflective continuing professional development audience. It is designed to encourage critical thinking, application of theory, critical reflection and analysis. The arguments in the book are grounded in the evidence base and current research is drawn upon to support these bringing the debates to life. Case study examples are peppered through the text to illustrate the issues under discussion and a global perspective is threaded throughout the book. Contemporary perspectives are considered throughout including changing technology and the use of social media in health communication.

Who should read it?

The primary audience for *Health Communication: Theoretical and Critical Perspectives* is a post-graduate audience and students in their final year of undergraduate programmes related to health, health promotion and public health. The book is also highly suitable for a variety of post-registration health and healthcare practitioners and any practitioner who has a role in health improvement. This will include post-graduate students in health promotion, public health, nursing including community nursing, health psychology and other health professionals. It may also include those studying, or working in, community development.

Overview of the book

The first part of the book outlines what we see as the three main disciplines contributing to health communication. In Part 1: Theoretical Perspectives, we critically explore relevant theory drawing on the three key disciplinary perspectives that are crucial for communicating health promotion and public health, namely education, communication and psychology. In this part of the book a range of theories are described, discussed, applied and critiqued with reference to the international research literature in health communication. The second section of the book Part 2: Key Topics is organized chapter by chapter around some contemporary topic areas in health communication. It looks at three key areas in turn: methods and media, social marketing and health literacy. The final section of the book Part 3: Issues and Challenges focuses on some of the broader challenges in health communication and in changing behaviour. There are three chapters in this part of the book. The first considers challenges in health communication and behaviour change. The second critically debates the politics of health communication and behaviour change. The final chapter in the book looks to the future in anticipation of what changes in society, technology and communication may have on how health is promoted through communication efforts. Each of the book's chapters is now briefly outlined in turn.

Chapter 2 – Communication Theory

Chapter 2 provides a critical overview of communication theories relating to health communication. Effective communication is central to any human encounter and is crucial in effecting changes in health promotion. The chapter provides a critical discussion of communication models underpinning health promotion practice. It explores one-way, top-down information transfer and two-way communication of health messages. It discusses the dialogical importance of communication that leads to empowerment and change in society. It then discusses the personal and interpersonal nature of health communication and the importance of knowledge and skills in communicating health messages, considering the different elements within the communication loop in a critical manner. The chapter takes a critical view of the health promoter as an effective communicator and an expert witness in health, challenging received assumptions and debating some ethical dilemmas in the context of environmental, social and cultural societal norms. Running through this chapter (and, indeed, the book as a whole) is a more complex discussion about power and empowerment, the scope for, and availability of, choice and control. As such Power Analysis is discussed as a way of considering the meaning of empowerment.

Chapter 3 – Educational Theory

This chapter provides the reader with an overview of the relation-ship between progressive educational theory and health promotion, highlighting what it is and why it may be of value to the professional practitioner. In defining progressive educational theory, it becomes clear that it is vital to health promotion – both in theory and in prac-tice – and is indeed key to achieving the social justice agenda that is championed in health promotion. Central to this is Freire's much maligned theory of empowerment and so, in a timely reappraisal, we evaluate his ideas to see if they are still relevant to professional practitioners today. Following a critical discussion which looks at the implications of Freire's empowerment theory, we introduce the progressive educational ideas of John Dewey and Martin Buber who provide alternative but complementary theories to empowerment that are worthy of consideration.

Chapter 4 – Psychological Theory

This chapter draws on theories of behaviour change from the dis-cipline of psychology. It outlines the key theoretical approaches to understanding the process of behaviour change and considers what the evidence is to support these. It draws on international research to examine the complexities of human behaviour and describe the key approaches which are taken. Key theories are briefly outlined, and then critiqued. These include the 'classic' major theories in this field such as the Health Belief Model, the Theory of Reasoned Action and the Theory of Planned Behaviour, the Trans-Theoretical Model and Protection Motivation Theory. The chapter then moves on to intro-duce and critique other innovations in behaviour change theory such as social psychological theory concerned with the influence of others, the notion of self-esteem and perceptions of control and two further specific theories – the Behavioural Ecological Model and the Theory of Triadic Influence. Throughout this chapter relevant research find-ings are drawn upon to illustrate key points and enhance the discus-sion, bringing theoretical features to life.

Chapter 5 – Methods and Media

This chapter discusses the methods and media used in communi-cating health messages. It will specifically look at mass media and related theory such as Diffusion of Innovation theory. Mass media can be a powerful agent for bringing about social change. However, it tends to be a one-way, top-down communication strategy which is often persuasive (even manipulative) and paternalistic. This chapter will critique popular methods of communication within health promotion such as TV and radio, art and drama, and emotional appeals as well as participatory approaches such as peer education. The evidence base and the effectiveness of these methods will be explored. It considers the use of media advocacy and narrowcasting as a way to influence policy change. The development of information communication technology has been rapid and profound over the past two decades. The use of electronic communications such as mobile phone technology, internet and social media as a channel for communicating health messages is increasingly popular. This chapter will therefore also critically analyse the development of electronic media as a communication method. It ends by considering some limitations of, and challenges in, health communication.

Chapter 6 – Social Marketing

This chapter provides an overview of social marketing, outlines what social marketing is and highlights how social marketing can be applied to health communication and health promotion. It reviews the literature on social marketing examining the relevance of it to health communication and establishing the strengths and weaknesses of social marketing as a strategy for health promotion. Taking a critical stance, this chapter explores the efficacy of social marketing and looks at how social marketing has been utilized in a variety of international contexts. It also examines the confusing/competing relationship of social marketing as a strategy to promote health linking to critical commentary elsewhere in this book about the use of mass media as a method for communicating health messages.

Chapter 7 – Health Literacy

In Chapter 7 we look at the increasingly important concept of health literacy in the field of health promotion and take a critical look at this evolving concept and its implications for effective health communication. We trace the historical origins and development of health literacy to reveal competing and divergent definitions, focusing in particular on the functional definition of health literacy which, arguably, since the millennium has come to dominate English-speaking nations. We evaluate the contribution of functional health literacy and note the limitations of an approach which, despite the rapid developments in global digital technology, still centres on basic competence in traditional literacies. Dependent upon organized systems of healthcare and tied to the power of the written word, we will show functional health literacy to be a peculiarly Western project ideally suited to positivist health frameworks which claim to evidence effectiveness in health promotion interventions. In response to calls for a more inclusive and critical form of health literacy, we explore other possibilities for a radical reconceptualization of health literacy: one that is grounded in informal adult education theories which empower communities to question, participate and act to deliver a critical experiential form of health literacy.

Chapter 8 – Challenges in Health Communication and Behaviour Change

This chapter takes a more critical approach to the concept of behaviour change and the issues and challenges that health promoters face in communicating health messages to a diverse population. It will outline the key challenges that exist adopting a more analytical approach to the notion of behaviour. It draws on the wider literature to consider what challenges are faced and how these might be overcome to promote better health outcomes. We therefore consider alternative ways of thinking about behaviour and behaviour change discussing ideas about 'health behaviours' in contrast with notions of 'social practices'. We critically examine communication issues relating to factors such as culture, gender and age, focusing on challenges arising from communicating with different groups of people in different contexts. The chapter critically considers process and structural barriers in communicating health messages. Finally it includes an appraisal of ethical issues in health communication such as those associated with dilemmas in persuasive and coercive communication, and the challenges that such methods pose to concerns within empowerment.

Chapter 9 – The politics of Health Communication and Behaviour Change

This chapter brings together a critical overview of the content covered thus far and highlights what we believe are some of the key political debates in health communication, debates that are central to health promotion considered as a more radical, social endeavour.

Taking a social constructionist perspective this chapter unpicks the notion of health communication as the route to behaviour change and challenges linear assumptions that this is the primary solution for improving health outcomes. Drawing on debates around individualism, agency and structure which are linked to concepts of citizenship and governmentality, it appraises the politics of health communication and behaviour change within the contemporary context of an increasingly neoliberal public health agenda.

Chapter 10 – Looking to the Future

This final chapter in the book begins by returning to the main themes of the book. It then discusses the mechanisms of global health communication followed by a consideration of changing technologies and the potential, but uncertain, futures these bring as well as the implications for health communication. A new paradigm is presented which reconstructs health behaviour as 'social theories of practice' and we argue for the use of critical perspectives and techniques in health communication. Finally, we put forward a challenge to competency frameworks.

Pedagogical features in health communication: theoretical and critical perspectives

In Chapters 2 to 9, there are four opportunities for reflection within each chapter provided at key stages in the discussion. At these points the reader is invited to engage in a task related to the content of the chapter. Each chapter also has suggestions for further reading with a short annotation about the nature of the text so that the reader can follow things up accordingly. The book contains case studies and international examples which aim to bring the issues under consideration to life. In addition, there are key insights provided which are labelled 'Implication for Practice' where it is intended that learning can be taken forward by the reader.

2
Communication Theory

Key aims

- To present a critical overview of key communication theory relevant to health communication
- To critically consider communication from a personal and interpersonal perspective
- To examine the concept of the 'expert' in health communication
- To critically consider the concepts of power and empowerment in relation to health communication

Introduction

This chapter critically discusses communication theories and models relating to health promotion practice. It examines the one-way, top-down transfer of health information and the two-way communication of health messages, promoting bottom-up (i.e. data driven) information processing, the dialogical importance of communication leading to empowering changes among specific audiences in particular and society in general. It looks at the importance of knowledge and skills in communicating health messages, discussing the different elements within the communication process in a critical manner. Thus it considers the concept of 'self' and the importance of self-awareness for the effective health communicator. The chapter explores the interaction and relationships between the health communicator, the public, policy makers and colleagues directly as well as indirectly, focusing on challenging the health professionals in practice and their assumptions as expert witnesses in health. Finally, it debates some of the inherent political and ethical dilemmas in communication as well as exploring the importance of social context in terms of environmental, societal and cultural norms.

Health promotion and communication

Communication about health is everywhere. It is hard to escape the constant messages about health that we are bombarded with on a daily basis. Messages are relayed via a variety of means such as through mobile phones, news articles, billboards, radio and television programmes, for example. Often such messages are in direct competition and at odds with lots of other types of message such as food advertising. Effective and appropriate communication is crucial in enabling changes for health improvement in today's information overloaded world. In health promotion and health communication we aim to work with individuals and communities to bring about sustainable changes and enable healthier choices. It is crucial, therefore, that we understand some of the key communication theories underpinning the process of communication in facilitating successful change. As discussed in Chapter 1, health promotion can be conceptualized as a social movement that brings about social justice in health (Cross et al., 2013). It therefore addresses health inequalities and the social determinants of health, focusing on the upstream approaches to health improvement (i.e. addressing the bridges and barriers to health/well-being rather than simply the downstream, treatment of illness/disease). Health communication is not just about designing credible health messages. It is about how a message is communicated effectively to individuals, groups and communities, enabling a bottom-up approach to behaviour changes; to policy makers or wider social and economic actors, effecting a policy change; and to colleagues on working collaboratively to facilitate change. As Anderson and Nishtar (2011: 9) state, 'because community attitudes are so central to individual behaviour, comprehensive public health initiatives, including legislative and health care approaches, must include a communication strategy that increases health literacy and tackles social norms. Thus, communication in all its forms has an unparalleled role in determining population attitudes and beliefs that can cultivate the perception that healthy living is a societal value rather than a personal choice.'

Health promotion as a 'discipline' interacts with other areas such as psychology, education, marketing, sociology and social policy, for example (Bunton and Macdonald, 2004). Within health promotion work and publications, much attention is given to methods of communication, design of health messages and, ultimately, to behaviour change. Communication theories have not received the same attention as other health promotion theories and models (Cross et al., 2013) yet, we would argue, they are crucial to health communication.

Communicating health: the development of communication theory

Understanding communication is important for all health professionals. In health promotion, we communicate to give and seek information, to develop understanding, provide advice, to teach and support, to socialize and to express our views. Good communication skills are essential to the effective delivery of a health communication message. A common assumption is that health messages are only considered to be effective when the audience has acted or responded to a message that ultimately aims to increase health goals (Corcoran, 2013). However, it is important to be critical about this. We need to consider whether the intended recipient has actually 'heard' the message but decided not to act on it, or whether they, in fact, do not have the resources to act even if they wanted to. In either case it is too simplistic to assume that the communication effort has simply been unsuccessful.

Simplistic parameters for success may lead to a disconnect between the valued outcomes of those seeking to improve health through communication efforts and those who are the intended beneficiaries. For example, it may appear that people do not listen. There is a common assumption that a change in people's knowledge and beliefs leads to a change in behaviour (Thompson and Kumar, 2011). Lee and Garvin's (2003) critique of health communication pointed out the problems with this assumption and the implications that information in health is largely linear, unidirectional and uncomplicated flowing from experts to individual. Individual level power and agency is seen as sufficient to improve health outcomes given the information provided, the assumption being that, if the message is well communicated, change will follow. Indeed, Fletcher (1973: 10) in *Communication in Medicine* viewed the purpose of communication in health as being to effect a change in the recipient's knowledge, attitudes and behaviour; more than just delivering a message. Although Fletcher did discuss the importance of feedback to check the effectiveness of the communication process, his focus was more on the recipients, the outcome of communication and the willingness of the information provider to realize that *'more may be learnt than taught'*. This perspective clearly privileges expert wisdom.

In many ways we have not come a lot further in the forty years since Fletcher's publication. The focus of many health communication interventions is often the people in receipt of health messages. This view suggests communication in health is top-down. As 'experts' we advise people on what is good for them and what they should be doing. The expectation is that the recipient changes as a result. Lee and Garvin (2003) see three key problems with this view, namely, the focus on the individual, expert knowledge being superior to lay perspectives and the one-way information transfer. They suggest that health professionals need to move beyond this monological information transfer towards dialogical information exchange. From the perspective of critical social theories (Patton, 2002) the power of experts and 'truth' over (supposedly) passive lay people ignores the social, cultural, environmental and structural barriers in behaviour change. Lee and Garvin argue (2003) for a dialogical information exchange approach to redirect the dominant approach of information transfer in health communication towards social relationships and context-oriented approaches, taking account of the agency of information recipients. Health information is not simply received, but thought about and acted upon (or not).

Communication theories – an overview

Communication as a discipline is relatively recent. The study of information transmission was only developed after the Second World War, the beginning of the mass communication period. Indeed, the focus on 'propaganda' in Nazi Germany, coupled with an emergent business model focus on marketing, shifted communication from art to science. The last fifty years have seen a great deal of development in the area of communication with the production of many powerful information communication technologies. The study of interpersonal communication has also become a key area of study. Early definitions of communication focused more on the mechanics of message exchange. More recently, our understanding of this has become more sophisticated and complex. Interpersonal communication adds yet more layers to it, about meaning, identity and relationship that are negotiated through direct face-to-face communication (Baxter and

Braithwaite, 2008). All of this has direct relevance to health promotion and health communication.

In health promotion, it is important to develop the skills for communication and to understand the process of transferring information from the sender ('health communicator') to the receiver (the public, policy makers, colleagues) to maximize the effectiveness of information transfer. Successful interventions are not just about the message recipients. They are also about the health promoters as well as the intervention itself. Bennett (1975: 3) defined communication as a 'process by which senders and receivers of messages interact in given social contexts' where the communicator is included and where there is an interaction. It is two-way traffic concerned with the exchange of meanings through a common set of symbols, a process involving the transmission of a 'coded' message between source and audience, 'a process in which participants create and share information with one another to reach a mutual understanding' (Rogers, 1995: 17). Having good communication skills and understanding the factors that influence the effectiveness of health messages is essential. We need to reflect on whether we are effective communicators rather than simply assume people will do what experts advise. This includes, for example, critically reflecting on the methods used, the design of these and how we measure success. We now consider developments in Communication Theories over the past seventy years, from the basic ideas of broadcasting messages to more complex interactions.

A basic model of communication

A basic version of the communication process has the message sender, the message and the receiver via a communication channel, and a feedback loop. In this model, to improve the effectiveness of health communication, we need to look at these components critically and the journey of the message that flows forward and backward from the sender through to the receiver, looking at the barriers that may arise at each stage of the journey – the communication process. Figure 2.1 and Box 2.1 (adapted from Cross et al., 2013) provide a simple way of looking at the issues within each component of the message journey.

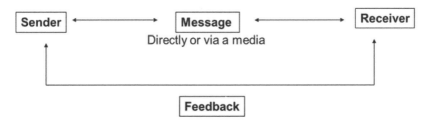

Figure 2.1 The message journey in the communication process (adapted from Cross et al., 2013)

Box 2.1 The components within the communication process (adapted from Cross et al., 2013)

Senders	Who we are and how we communicate. Our communication skills – verbal, non-verbal, written. Do we listen to the message receivers? How self-aware are we as communicators?
Messages	Is our message simple or complicated? Is it appropriate, easy to understand? How do we 'code' our message?
Channels	What communication methods did we choose: mass media, interpersonal communication? The environment where the message was transmitted.
Receivers	Who are the audience? What is their literacy level, their state of mind, their views, their beliefs and attitudes, their social and living environment?

Communication theories – from traditional linear to complex

For those who subscribe to a top-down approach to communication in health, the traditional linear transmission model of communication fits well. Lasswell's (1948) Formula of One-Way Communication is a classic model of how communication is the transfer of information from source to recipients. This early model of communication described the process as 'who says what, to whom, in which channel, with what effect?' It represents early understandings of communication where there is simply an intention to influence and where communication is viewed as a persuasive process. The purpose of effecting a change within the recipient is implicit. The primary purpose is to transmit a message and for the message to have an effect (McQuail and Windahl, 1993). In that post-war era the persuasive power of mass communication, particularly marketing, was very prominent. Although Lasswell was criticized for the lack of a feedback loop, top-down communication symbolized power and, as such, was well-suited to an era of fascist regimes. Feedback was not important; indeed, feedback is missing in this formula. Although the model was developed more than sixty years ago, it still forms the contemporary basis for much of the study, and execution, of mass communication.

Shannon-Weaver's Model of Communication (1949) is another linear, one-way transmission model from the same period. This again presents communication as a one-way process of information transfer with an added element of 'noise'. The model was developed from Shannon's work in telecommunication, but has been used analogically by behavioural and linguistic scientists. The noise in Shannon-Weaver's model was originally about the *literal* noise in the transmission of messages in telecommunication, namely interference inhibiting the transmission process. The *metaphorical* noise in Shannon-Weaver's model refers to factors that influence the communication process. Hargie and Dickson (2004) view 'noise' as either the intrusive sound occurring *externally* in the environment and social context or *internally* through the life experience of the individual, for example, ethnic and cultural choices of words or expression. There are many factors influencing the effectiveness of communication in health which can originate at source; channel, receiver or context. These 'noises' should be key considerations in health communication, for example, poor readability (Hamilton and Chou, 2014). Hamilton and Chou (2014) see this as an opportunity rather than a barrier to effective communication. They looked at noise generated in the personal, community and institutional context and see it as essential background aspects of interpersonal encounters which needs to be recognized, identified and managed, arguing that this helps practitioners to rethink effective communication and appropriate interventions. As with Lasswell's formula, feedback in Shannon-Weaver's model is also missing. However, feedback is vitally important. We learn from feedback in order to improve and to assess if the communication process has been effective. Feedback therefore plays a central role in social interaction and successful social outcomes (Hargie and Dickson, 2004). Crucially, classic communication models such as Lasswell's and Shannon-Weaver's do not take into account social context and the different meanings that can be interpreted by the message receivers (Hartley, 1999).

The traditional, linear, one-way models of communication are described by Clampitt (2001) as the 'arrow approach'. Clampitt criticized these models for being simplistic and not reflecting the richness and complex dynamics in human communication (Rogers, 1986). Corcoran (2013) argues that human communication is cyclical and, increasingly, theoretical models have come to mean two-way communication (Kiger, 2004). Following on from Lasswell, Shannon-Weaver and many other linear models of one-way communication, Osgood and Schramm (in Schramm, 1954) developed a *circular model* of communication. They thought of communication as a cyclic process. Messages are passed between coders and encoders (senders and receivers) with no end-point to the process. There is an exchange of information forwards and backwards. The sender becomes receiver in the feedback process, and the receiver becomes sender. Both interpret each other's messages and both give and receive feedback to and from each other. Clampitt (2001) described this as the 'circuit approach' to communication. The premise is that we act as simultaneous coder and decoder when sending and receiving messages and interpret information as we receive it.

Osgood and Schramm (Schramm, 1954) also implied an equal relationship between sender and receiver in communication exchange (McQuail and Windahl, 1993). However, as health promoters, the 'experts' in delivering health messages to the public, we have to consider our own assumptions and behaviour and the nature of the relationship between ourselves and the people with whom we work. The power balance between health promoters and clients can easily be overlooked and needs to be addressed. We discuss this in more detail later in this chapter and in Chapter 9. The social exchange in communication can also be seen in Hartley's (1999) Simple Model of Interpersonal Communication, where the social context is important. The social identity and perception of both sender and receiver feature in Hartley's model. The assumption is that our mental and cognitive processes shape our actions and how we communicate. As with Osgood and Schramm's circular model, the cyclic, two-way communication models are different to the linear models of one-way communication which do not provide room for interpretation or clarification.

Within health promotion literature, Hubley's (2004) communication model clearly shows the different components within the
two-way communication loop in health communication activities.
Different actors/characteristics within each component of the communication loop will shape the effectiveness of the communication
process. Feedback provides a link to complete the communication
circuit for the message source (the health promoter) and the message
receiver (the public). This is a way to check the accuracy of information provision and a form of evaluation of the effectiveness of health
promotion activities which may promote evidence for practice.

Green et al. (2015) present a more comprehensive communication model developed from telecommunications, showing the communication process and the reciprocal relationship between message
source and receiver (see Figure 2.2). The model shows how messages
are encoded by the sender. In health communication we use different
ways and means to communicate messages. By using *symbolic* codes,
we can show for example the devastating effect of gonorrhoea using a
picture; the effect of a child dying from a car accident, or the effects
of second-hand smoke. By using *iconic* codes, we can show we care
about people dying of breast cancer by donning a pink ribbon, or in
the case of HIV/AIDS, by a red ribbon. We can use *enactive* codes
by involving people in some kind of activities, for example, Race for
Life. Our non-verbal signs show the sincerity of our intentions. Our
message is then interpreted and decoded by our receivers. It may be
stored in their memory and motivate them to change at some point.
Successful communication occurs when the receiver's interpretation
exactly matches the communicator's intended message (Green et
al., 2015). The effectiveness is dependent on the receiver accurately
decoding and interpreting the message and motivation to change.
This is the challenge!

Implication for Practice 1

It is important to be explicit if, and how, you seek feedback from your
intended recipients on the health communication interventions that you
are engaged in. When designing a communication campaign, it is essential
to consider the different components within the communication process.

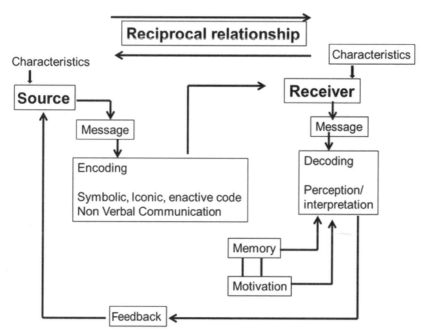

Figure 2.2   Communication Model (Green et al., 2015, p. 313)

From communication models to conversations

As alluded to already, communication is not simply about information transfer. Even the more complex communication models have
their limitations. It is therefore useful to also think about communication as *conversation*. Ordinary conversation is not simply about
strategic planning and technical models. It is person to person and it
is personal.

The methods in communicating health messages can be broadly
divided into two categories: (1) mass communication where messages are indirectly and widely communicated to recipients via media
where direct interaction is missing and (2) interpersonal communication where direct interaction between senders and recipients occurs.
While focusing on these two categories we realize that there are other
forms of communication. For example, intrapersonal communication
can also be important, where internal communication occurs within
oneself, internal discourse involving thinking, reflecting and analysing; self-talk . . . how we make sense of incoming messages internally,
based on our background, our beliefs, values and attitudes.

Most health communication literature focuses on messages and recipients – the sender is seen as an objective professional looking down, trying to bring about strategic change, scientific, uninvolved and impersonal. This section focuses primarily on the message sender and *direct two-way interpersonal communication* (though we will also make reference to intrapersonal communication). Characteristics of the message recipients in the communication process are explored in more depth in Chapter 4.

Hargie and Dickson (2004) argue that communication is transactional, inevitable, purposeful, multi-dimensional and irreversible. Interpersonal communication is a spontaneous, non-mediated interaction. It involves social interaction between two or more parties. Information, meaning and feelings are shared by exchanging verbal and non-verbal messages. Baxter and Braithwaite (2008) looked at three different approaches to interpersonal communication in healthcare: (1) *individual-centred* theories, a cognitive activity focusing on how individuals plan, produce and process messages; (2) *interaction-centred* theories focusing on interaction between people; and (3) *relationship-centred* theories which focus on the relationships between people. We would argue that the process of communicating health messages to another person or persons must involve all three approaches as described by Baxter and Braithwaite (2008) namely, the individual taking the initiative to communicate; the interaction; and, if there is interaction, there must be some kind of relationship.

The two common factors in interpersonal communication are people and relationships. It should be interactive and relational and it should always be two-way. Good social skills are necessary in effective interpersonal communication (Hartley, 1999; Hargie and Dickson, 2004). The process also takes place within, and is influenced by, context, environment and social structure. In discussing interpersonal communication, Hartley (1999) subdivided social context into physical and social environment; social and cultural norms, social rules and social relationships. We will focus on the communicator as the person initiating the health communication process.

Being reflective and self-aware is crucial in health communication. This is, obviously, also where interpersonal and intrapersonal processes overlap. Critical reflection is a useful tool to evaluate, learn from and adapt for practice. Our communication methods can be very important in influencing our clients' choices. But how often do we consider our own communication style and skills? How aware are we of how we communicate health messages to others? How effective are we? Knowledge is fundamental at every stage of the communication process (Hargie and Dickson, 2004). The knowledge and power of the expert can be overpowering. The authority of the message source is one of the determining factors that may affect the receivers' acceptance of the message. On the one hand, the credibility of the information source seems important in health communication. On the other, people are experts by experience in their own lives which can be ignored by both the expert sender and the recipients themselves. On a superficial level, as in both Hubley's (2004) and Green et al.'s (2015) models of communication, sender characteristics such as gender, age, appearance and so forth may influence the acceptability of the message. On a deeper level, we need to be aware of where the expertise actually lies.

The cultural understanding and appropriateness may facilitate and enhance the acceptability of health messages. Conversely, lack of understanding of an individual's culture (as well as the awareness of our own culture) may hinder the delivery of health messages resulting in unintended outcomes. Audience segmentation is a principle in social marketing and is an important first step in developing targeted health communication programmes. Culture can be an important audience segmentation variable (see Chapter 6 for more detail). Similarly, epidemiological data can be useful in exploring the relevance of health communication messages to specific groups of people. Indeed, categorizing people into different groups can be powerful in terms of understanding different groups' specific needs, although it may result in stereotyping which can have a negative, detrimental effect in communication (Hargie and Dickson, 2004).

Kreuter and McClure (2004) argue that operational definitions and good models of cultural sensitivity and cultural appropriateness in health are lacking. Culture is generally viewed as being the values, beliefs, norms and practices of a social group. However, this perspective can potentially be limiting. When developing health campaigns, diversity and culture should be taken into account (IOM, 2002). Kreuter and McClure (2004) looked at the role of culture in health communication. They studied the source, message and channel factors in culturally appropriate health communications. McGuire's (1989) Communication/Persuasion model presented five input variables in health communication planning – source, message, channel, receiver and destination. This has similarities with Lasswell's (1948) formula – who, says what, through which channel, to whom, with what effects. Source credibility such as expertise and trustworthiness can increase the acceptability of the message. Demographic similarities, attitudinal similarities such as values and beliefs may also increase the credibility of the message, adding to the appeal of evidence-based messages when they reflect the social and cultural world of the audience.

In health communication, the people that we work with may make the same assumptions as we do about our expertise. We may subconsciously fall into the belief that we are here to advise or to provide information perpetuating an 'expert knows best' agenda. Of course, we may indeed possess some knowledge about health. However, we are not, and can never be, experts of other people's lived experience and the economic, environmental and social aspects of their lives. Our behaviour and actions depend on various aspects of our social identity. Humanistic psychologists, such as Rogers, have studied the concept of 'self' in depth (Rogers, 1969). Illeris (2014: 37) described self as the 'mental centre of the individual and its self-understanding, self-confidence and self-realization'. Our own reasoning, emotions and conscience inform important beliefs about ourselves which we then relate to others. To be communicatively competent and to become better communicators, it is important to be aware of ourselves and how we present ourselves.

Most obviously, we communicate verbally and, of course, often also communicate through other means such as written messages or perhaps sign language for people with a hearing impairment. But in a direct one-to-one communication, or one-to-small-group communication, we communicate our views and attitudes via our body language, sometimes in conflict with what we actually say which may overshadow it. Green et al. (2015) described this as non-verbal leakage which may convey lack of genuineness or empathy. In fact, only 7 per cent of our face-to-face message is communicated by the words we choose; the rest is transmitted non-verbally. And of this 93 per cent, 38 per cent is communicated through our vocal tones and 55 per cent through facial expressions (British Institute of Learning Disability, 2005). Our motives, attitudes, personality, emotions, age, gender, culture, context, our values all impact on the way we communicate (Hargie and Dickson, 2004). Non-verbal communication such as body language, facial expressions, eye contact, tone of voice and personal space can transmit unintended messages. The strength of our actual communication is clearer and stronger (positively or negatively) than we may realize (Kiger, 2004).

The Johari Window (Box 2.2) is useful in helping us to better understand human interaction. It is a psychological tool created by Luft and Ingham (1955) which can help to improve self-awareness, promote communicative competence. The window is a representation of ourselves. Handy (1999) views it as a house with windows and

Box 2.2 The Johari Window (adapted from Handy, 1999)

	Known to self	Unknown to self
Known to others	1	2
Unknown to others	3	4

walls. Room 1 is an open space where we and others share the same knowledge. In Room 2 is what others know about us but we do not see ourselves – our 'blind' self. Room 3 is our private space containing that which we do not want others to see. Room 4 is a mysterious place that nobody knows – the 'unconscious' self.

Being self-aware and being reflective help us to have a better understanding of ourselves and thus to improve our communication skills. This is important both in interpersonal communication and in intrapersonal communication. When we are open, we allow others to understand our intentions. Through feedback from others, we can know more about ourselves. Through self-disclosure, we let people know more about us. Being aware of our own strengths and weaknesses can help us to understand our position, our arguments as we see them, our values and our beliefs. We become aware of how we communicate and can become better communicators. It also challenges the power relationship between the health promoters and the people whom we work with. An open and honest relationship may facilitate the co-construction of health. For example, if the health promoter has a strong view on a gender issue or disability issue, being reflective and self-aware help us to be reflexive, empathetic, not to impose our view on others in a judgemental manner.

Transactional analysis (TA) – see Box 2.3 – is an approach developed by Berne (1964) that examines human interaction. It is a psychological interpretation of how and why we act when interacting with others. Berne (1964) draws on Freudian psychodynamic theory and identified three ego states or observable personalities within every individual – parent, adult and child. Although we are not using TA as an interpersonal communication model nor do we intend to analyse an individual communicator's ego state or their behaviour, it is useful to understand and be aware of the way we act when we are communicating with others. For example, do we speak like a controlling parent in a paternalistic manner when we give advice on certain health issues such as smoking and drinking alcohol, or do we speak with a strong emotion and in a child-like manner?

Box 2.3 Transactional Analysis (adapted from Berne, 1964)

Parent	Nurturing, Controlling	Feel and behave in ways learnt from mother, father, teacher etc. It involves taking responsibility or assuming authority.
Adult	Rational	Observe, collect data, think, weigh probable outcomes of alternative course, make decisions.
Child	Feeling, Intuiting, Adapting	Feel and behave typically as a child. You experience strong feelings and emotions, create, have fun, adapt to or feel bad about the demands of more powerful people.

As health promoters, we aim to empower people and enable them to make choices that they believe in, that work for them and that they can adhere to. However, a 'parenting' educational approach can make the assumption that 'I am ok but you are not ok', arguably assuming a deficit position (see Box 2.4). Whether you are a controlling parent or nurturing parent, as seen in Harris's (2004) description of the orientations we adopt towards other people, the outcome is the same. Power lies with the health communication expert who knows 'best'. Conversely an empowerment approach starts from the perspective that 'I am ok, you are ok'. This reflects a negotiated, adult relationship, the co-construction of knowledge and dialogue, working together as equal partners in the process.

Box 2.4 I'm OK – you're OK (adapted from Harris, 2004)

I'm OK – You're OK	fine with yourself and accept others
I'm OK – You're not OK	uncomfortable with yourself (superficially 'okay', but actually in denial) but disown it and reflect on others' limitations
I'm not OK – You are OK	feel sorry for yourself and think others doing better
I'm not OK – You're not OK	unhappy about yourself and negative towards others

Implication for Practice 2
Good communication skills in health communication practice are essential because of the direct implications they have on the effectiveness of interventions. It is important to consider how you communicate in practice, to be aware of your own strengths and weakness, your non-verbal leakage and to consider what position you adopt in the relationship with the people you work with (expert? co-constructor of knowledge? facilitator?).

Theoretical models and personal interactions: the importance of power analysis

As the preceding section makes clear, human communication is more than simple, linear, mechanical models. Communication is complex. Increasingly words like 'empowerment' are used to make it rational and personal. However, the term 'empowerment' can be slippery and vague (Woodall et al., 2012). The over-use and misuse of the term can lead to it being perceived cynically, with diminished meaning (Laverack, 2013). Such terms have, themselves, also become professionalized (Forrest et al., 2013; Beresford et al., 2011). Often, communities (of locality, experience or identity) are cynical that words are manipulated by powerful people (sometimes professionals). For example, those in power can change the meaning of what is said – 'independence' to mean having to do everything by yourself, rather than having control over decisions that shape your life (Forrest et al., 2013)! This example of 'power-over', as described by Laverack (2013), can seem quite subtle but be very real.

People are empowered when they are able to influence decisions about their lives. They already have the potential to make decisions. Usually it has been taken away or is not supported (e.g. by those with power). Our role in health promotion and health communication is to build bridges and remove barriers to help people achieve fundamental human rights, civil rights and entitlements (WHO, 1986). Laverack (2013) sees the redistribution of power, transforming unequal power relationship within and between societies, as the key to addressing health inequalities. Historically, disciplines such as community development (Barr et al., 2001) have recognized the complex and ambivalent role of professionals in empowering communities. They recognize the role of professionals in supporting people, while not leaving communities as passive recipients of professional ideas. The same issues are relevant for communication theories, health and empowerment. So here, we would like to set the scene for the use of the word 'empowerment' in good communication.

There are many societal power theories and some are very similar. One particular framework (which has been used in a number of programmes by organizations such as the Carnegie Foundation, the Joseph Rowntree Charitable Trust, the Joseph Rowntree Foundation and the Institute for Development Studies) is Power Analysis (Gaventa, 2006; Hunjan and Keophilavong, 2010). Central to their framing of 'empowerment' is the idea of the Power Cube. They triangulate and critique power according to a number of dimensions (see Box 2.5).

Thus, empowerment in health promotion happens when we communicate at the level appropriate to people's lives and at the level where change is needed and likely to happen. This framework is honest about different types of power, recognizing the power already within communities to make changes or 'power with' as described

Box 2.5 Dimensions of Power

Level	Power is exercised at many different levels – international, national, regional or local. It is important to address power at the appropriate levels. Where do people operate? Where does change need to happen?
Forms	There are many different forms of power. *Visible* power – the power that different groups or communities themselves have; *Invisible* power – (e.g.) oppressive stereotypes that hold communities back; *Hidden* power – vested interests, usually in the background. Who needs to be in the conversation? Who needs to change?
Spaces	There are different types of spaces where power is exercised. *Closed* spaces where communities are excluded; *Invited* spaces where communities are invited – these can be *genuine* or *manipulated* spaces; *Claimed* spaces where communities are, where they themselves exercise power, where their ownership is unambiguous. Is the space authentic or fake?

by Laverack (2013), but it is also honest about the different levels of power, for example globalization, which can act against change but which, as individuals, we can do little by ourselves to reshape.

Health promotion is a discipline of empowerment. This means that we should not simply work in a top-down approach in health communication. An empowerment model of health promotion is about removing barriers, enabling person-centred decision-making. We are clear that we need to engage our clients in what we do. However, we need to be aware of how this takes place and minimize paternalistic, manipulative and coercive means. Maibach and Parrott (1995) purport that health communication is a goal-oriented activity focused on the message receivers that aims to influence change. Herein lies a dilemma. We may say the purpose of communication is to empower the individual or the public in their decision-making about their health. We would argue that health promoters can, indeed, use an empowerment approach to enable an informed decision-making process. But often this boils down to trying to influence change or telling people what the healthy option is. We provide information in the hope that people will choose what we think is right (based on evidence?). When facing poverty and social inequality, the ability and capacity to make affordable healthy choices can be limited. 'Good' choices also depend on values and cultural background. For example, a vegetarian diet may be seen as a healthy option in the Western world but lack credibility in a culture where eating meat is a sign of affluence. Similarly, an increase in weight in middle-class groups may be viewed as unhealthy in some cultures but desirable in others due to associations with prosperity.

The right and ability to make choices is seen as a good thing in a modern democratic society. This is particularly true in public health, based on the principles in the Ottawa Charter (WHO, 1986) of collaborating, enabling and empowering. However, in practice, the process of decision-making is often complex. Hence, making choices often means making a decision based on availability and restrictions within your personal life and family commitments. Choice for many people really means that there is no choice, but that they have to take what is available under the circumstances because of social and environmental barriers they are facing. In 'The Paradox of Choices' Schwartz (2004) argues that people often do not have a choice or, in fact, have too many choices. There are inherent ethical concerns in health communication such as, for example, using persuasive means, manipulating emotions and restricting control and choice. We discuss ethics in more depth in Chapter 8.

Hubley and Copeman with Woodall (2013) see health promotion as a continuum of activities from coercion, through persuasion, to empowerment. The punitive approach of coercion is easily distinguished. However, the line between persuasion and empowerment is more ambiguous. In health education, communication is a planned process (Kiger, 2004). Health education can, indeed, be seen as persuasion, a top-down approach to educate, persuade and shape people's behaviour. Some may see this as empowering. We provide information, seeking to develop an individual's decision-making skills, empowering people to decide what is good for them in their circumstances (Green, 2008).

In theory, persuasion and empowerment are quite different. There is no ambiguity between 'seeking to influence people' and 'helping people to develop decision-making skills and confidence to bring about changes'. Yet, theory is one thing, practice another. When we provide 'evidence-based' information to clients, are we selective? What evidence do we prioritize? How credible is the evidence? What tone of voice do we use? How aware are we of our body language? Do our non-verbal language, manner, attitude, body language tell the same story? When we say 'it's your choice', are we aware of the tone of voice we use? Do we understand our client's situation? Do we treat them as equals and active agents of change? Do they have the autonomy and the agency to act and make free choices? Power, credibility and attractiveness are three characteristics of the message-sender in trying to influence others and this links to social influence. Social influencing is when one person's actions have a causal effect on the outcomes or life events of another (Dickson et al., 1993). We are more likely to be influenced by people with charisma and people we like (Ajzen, 1992).

For some, persuasion limits empowerment and choice. Others believe in justified persuasion – steering in a helpful direction – when the evidence is strong (Hubley and Copeman with Woodall, 2013). Communication models can seem rational and scientific, with the professional being equally rational and guided by knowledge and research evidence. However, in practice, the line between persuasion and empowerment can be rather fine. It may even be dangerous when persuasion becomes manipulation (Cross et al., 2013). In health communication we do have an agenda – we want to promote health and effect change. We design health communication interventions and campaigns, choosing the best communication methods we think are appropriate for having the maximum impact.

Crucially, we need to be aware of the power we have over the people whom we work with. The source-receiver relationship can lead to an imbalance of power (Green et al., 2015). We may be in a very powerful position that we may not realize or that we may intentionally or unintentionally make use of. Laverack (2009) discussed the different types of power in public health work. Health 'experts' are often in an authoritative position, holding 'expert power' with 'legitimate power' as well as 'information power'. We may also use 'coercive power', the authority to punish if people break the law for example, by not wearing seat belts or smoking in public. We can also reward people with praise – 'reward power'. We can use other people's stories to support our causes for example, celebrities, global sports personalities or famous actors – 'reference power'.

Empowering an individual is about developing autonomous thinking, and we will discuss a range of education theories in more depth in Chapter 4. For the present, it is worth noting a few issues in relation to choice, education and construction of knowledge that are important in health communication. According to Mezirow (1997) in adult education, autonomous thinking is essential for the productive and responsible worker in the twenty-first century in a collaborative context, so that they are aware and critical in assessing assumptions, adapt to change, exercise critical judgement and flexibly engage in effective collaborative decision-making. Education is about developing learners' ability to construct their own meaningful reality which is key to empowerment enabling decision-making (Dewey, 1916; Freire, 1972). Effective communication is important for learning. It is learning itself that is responsible for change (Green et al., 2015). People are not passive recipients of information. We interpret and make sense of the world as we see it. From a social constructivist's point of view, we construct our own reality (see Chapter 9 for further discussion). Education is a process of co-construction of knowledge. A two-way communication process, as described in Osgood and Schramm's circular communication model, provides the opportunities for social interaction when both sender and receiver interpret and give feedback on each other's messages. Social interaction is important in knowledge construction and skill development (Vygotsky, 1978). Learning is a social process and discourse is central to making meaning. Interaction and participation encourage deeper learning (Mezirow, 1997). Mezirow's transformative learning is about changing one's frame of reference and critical reflection is important in the transformation process. We learn through critical thinking, communication and critical reflection as well as through others' experiences.

Implication for Practice 3

Being aware of the power we hold over people in practice is important. It is essential to consider how you engage in practice with people. Are your efforts and actions persuasive, coercive or manipulative or are they concerned with empowering control and choice?

Communication is complex. We will end this chapter by asking you to reflect on your own experiences. We said health communication is a goal-oriented activity (Maibach and Parrott, 1995). We use different methods to communicate health messages – sometimes one-way mass communication, sometimes two-way direct face-to-face discussion. Communication models see communication as a rational and technical process. The health communicator's goal is to prompt active thought among a passive audience. An active audience involved and engaged will actively seek, attend and process messages. Engagement can be enhanced, for example, by presenting messages in an unusual manner such as comics, drama, the use of specific language; positive image can provoke and trigger active thought and encourage the audience to process the incoming information – a bottom-up information processing process (Maibach and Parrott, 1995). We aim to motivate people, enable and empower, encourage bottom-up information processing where audiences consider health messages actively, interpret the meaning of messages and make the right choice for their lives.

Implication for Practice 4

Choosing an appropriate method for your health communication campaign is an important aspect of health promotion practice. Two-way communication seems more robust and effective, with an interactive process that refines knowledge, because of the feedback gained. However, the choice depends on the health topic and the target population. For example, one-way mass communication might be a better way to reach out to and empower some groups.

Summary of key points

This chapter has provided a critical overview of communication theory. Specifically it has:

- presented an overview of key communication theories relevant to health communication
- considered communication from a personal and interpersonal perspective
- examined the concept of the 'expert' in health communication
- considered the concepts of power and empowerment in relation to health communication

Reflection 1 – Reflecting on your experience, do you think you are an effective communicator? Are you aware of how you communicate with others? What are your strengths and weaknesses? Perhaps ask a close friend whom you can trust and will tell you the truth for some feedback on how you communicate.

Reflection 2 – Was there a time when you may have 'unconsciously' presented yourself as a parent when you delivered a health message, taking a paternalistic approach in imparting your knowledge, a top-down, medical or educational approach? Was there a time when you presented yourself in an emotional manner, perhaps getting annoyed (acting like a child) with your clients when they did not follow your instructions or did not agree with your 'logical' arguments ('It's your choice' 7 per cent message *(sighs and shrugs shoulders dismissively)* 93 per cent meaning)? Have you always behaved and acted as an adult and treated others as adults, as an equal partner when you communicate with your clients, taking a dialogical approach that empowers the clients, taking an authentic empowerment approach?

Reflection 3 – When you offer your clients choices, do you think they really have a choice? Have you considered their predicament and put yourself in their shoes when making a choice?

Reflection 4 – The health communicator's goal is to prompt active thought in an, at times, passive audience. Reflecting on your experience, how would you engage those who are not interested in health messages? How might their interest be motivated?

Further reading

Cross, R., O'Neil, I. and Dixey, R. (2013) Communicating health. In Dixey, R. (ed.) (2013) *Health Promotion: Global Principles and Practice.* CABI.
Chapter 4 'Communicating Health' is a very useful chapter that gives you a summary and an insight into communicating health messages.
Green, J., Tones, K., Cross, R. and Woodall, J. (2015) *Health Promotion: Planning and Strategies.* 3rd edn. London: Sage.
Chapter 7 'Education for Health' is really helpful. It looks at the communication process linking to education theories, persuasion and attitude change. The communication model in this chapter (Figure 2.2) is from the chapter in this book.
Lee, R. G. and Garvin, T. (2003) Moving from information transfer to information exchange in health and health care. *Social Science and Medicine,* 56, 449–64.
This article, although a little older, is very good, discussing how health professionals communicate health messages and the problems with one-way communication. It explains the need for a two-way communication in health practice.

3
Educational Theory

Key aims

- To define the key features of progressive educational theory and practice, outlining its relationship to health communication and health promotion
- To locate Freirean empowerment theory as part of the progressive tradition in education and explore the implications of a Freirean approach to health communication in health promotion
- To reappraise the contribution of empowerment theory and highlight the challenges associated with its current application in health communication and health promotion
- To introduce the progressive educational ideas of John Dewey and Martin Buber with the aim of resolving the challenges associated with empowerment theory in relation to health communication and health promotion in practice

Introduction

This chapter gives an overview of the relationship between progressive educational theory and health promotion, highlighting what it is and why it is important to professional practice. Here, we identify a core set of values and beliefs which uniquely define its purpose and methods, revealing progressive education to be radically different from mainstream practice – but in tune with the transformative agenda of health promotion. Taking a critical stance, this chapter will review the key aspects of one particular theory that has come to dominate health promotion – Freire's theory of empowerment

– and will explore the implications of this theory for health communication in practice. This chapter presents a timely reappraisal of Freire's contribution to health promotion while highlighting some challenges associated with the approach. So other theories from the progressive tradition will be considered: more specifically, the ideas of John Dewey and Martin Buber, which complement and enable a more insightful, practical understanding of Freirean empowerment theory.

Overview of the relationship between progressive educational theory and health promotion

Practitioners who think of themselves as *health promoters* rather than *educators* might be asking what educational theory has to do with health communication in promoting health. We believe quite a lot because, above all else, it is the *educative* process that has the potential to change health behaviours. In contrast to information giving, the educational process is a dynamic, enabling process that, at its best, involves a mutual exchange of knowledge as well as active opportunities to build new or existing knowledge. Green et al. (2015: 25) suggest that effective health education has the strongest potential to bring about long-term sustainable change because it

> may result in the development of cognitive capabilities such as the acquisition of factual information, understanding and insights. It may also provide skills in problem-solving and decision-making and the formation of new beliefs. It might also result in the clarification of existing values . . . and, quite frequently, in attitude change.

That said, this does not mean that all forms of education should be regarded as equally useful or suited to the purposes of health communication, particularly the radical agenda in the 'militant wing' of health promotion which claims to work ethically to advance the practices of advocacy, equity and most importantly – empowerment. A brief study of educational theory makes this plain by bringing into view the hidden ideological structures that operate within education, revealing different and competing conceptualizations. A greater understanding of educational theory also exposes the values that underpin these differing approaches and how those values, in turn, inform the curricula and methods which are used to realize a specific educational purpose. Thus, if the purpose of health education is to effect a change in values and attitudes as we suggest, we must look to progressive educational theory.

Bound by similar commitments to the radical health promoter, progressive educationalists have certain ideas about education that tie them to a social justice agenda. As a result, progressive education tends to focus on the underutilized *affective* domain in learning which deals with a person's feelings and emotions, rather than on the cognitive learning functions that deal with thinking, reasoning and evaluation (Wormeli, 2015). Consequently, progressive educators are primarily concerned with creating non-threatening, non-competitive participatory learning environments where positive relationships can be nurtured – not just between the teacher and student body – but between students by advancing the values of cooperation, support and friendship.

Defining the purpose and practices of progressive education

The ultimate purpose of progressive education is to *enable* and once able, it follows that individuals can self-actualize (Maslow, 1970) and, as individuals or as members of a collective, participate fully and actively in the ever widening circles of family, community and society. This is a transformative process and it is precisely this quality which the health promoter seeks to replicate in practice. However, capturing a singular and stable definition of transformative education is problematic and this is reflected in the literature as the underpinning philosophy and practices associated with it are informed by many disciplines and sub-disciplines (Hoggan, 2016). Precise locations of practice are equally challenging to pin down since a diversity of professionals – including health promoters – now make use of transformational educational theory. Further difficulty arises because of the essential dynamism of transformational education: a bespoke experience that is continuously shaped within a unique democratic framework, reflecting anew the motivations and abilities of those who participate in it.

Despite numerous and shifting definitions, transformative education and its many referents such as 'socially purposeful education' or 'community education' *does* form a distinct branch of educational practice recognizable both by its methods and purpose. Unlike individualist forms of education (both formal and non-formal) which rest on competition, competency and credit, transformative education is essentially a *moral* enterprise where knowledge is pursued collectively and informally to gain a deeper understanding of life – a necessary prerequisite to becoming an active citizen – or agent in public life. This concept of education is political as well as moral, and is part of an old tradition that can be traced back to Greek Antiquity and in particular to the influential ideas of Aristotle (2004) and Cicero (2001) who all understood learning (acquiring knowledge) to be a relational *process*.

This process principally demands two things of educators: firstly, the ability to care genuinely about the well-being and futures of those they work with and secondly, in addition to their command of the subject, skill in fostering dialogue in the form of Socratic questioning (http://infed.org/mobi/plato-on-education). Socratic questioning is a very specific type of dialogue which purposefully explores (and tests) the boundaries of knowledge. What is most prized in this reciprocal educative relationship is the development of 'criticality' – that is to say, curious and questioning minds. In transformational learning the notion of knowledge as fixed or even entirely knowable is rejected, making standardized curricula and the transfer of facts of little educational value.

Transformational education theory and health communication

Health promoters use communication as a tool to effect change at an individual, community and societal level and therefore we ought to be interested in progressive, transformational educational theories. Underpinned by radically different values to those operating in mainstream education, these theories can offer valuable insights about 'what works' especially among people and communities that are disadvantaged and disenfranchised (www.learningandwork.org. uk). 'What works' is an altogether different approach to education that is based on an alternative pedagogy that supports a broad set of dynamic practices reflecting a deep, non-negotiable commitment to global as well as local democracy, and social justice. In practising this form of education, values appear on the surface rather than being hidden and are tangible in the relations fostered between students and tutors. These values are also evident in the curricula, teaching materials and methods which necessarily embrace the lived experience of students. Unlike formal and non-formal educational settings, the educator works with people cooperatively to negotiate collectively the ways in which to build knowledge so that they will ultimately be enabled by their learning to *act*. This form of educational praxis is demanding and has implications for the professional practitioner because as Giroux highlighted,

> Radical pedagogy requires non-authoritarian social relationships that support dialogue and communication as indispensable for questioning the meaning and nature of knowledge and peeling away the hidden structures of reality. (Giroux, 1981: 133)

This radical transformative agenda stands in direct opposition to instrumental ideas that shape much of mainstream education today, privileging instead the purpose and methods of the old tradition which – then as now – depend upon a 'vital informality' (O'Rourke, 1995). Steeped in the personal experience-based reflections of the participants, this type of education – aided by skilled facilitation – critically probes existential questions about the nature of social reality and therefore by implication, inequality. Johnson (1979) defines this as 'really useful knowledge' which is

> [A] knowledge of everyday circumstances, including a knowledge of why you were poor, why you were politically oppressed and why through the force of social circumstance, you were the kind of person you were, your character misshapen by a cruel competitive world. (Education Group, 1981, cited in Avis, 2004:167)

Based on an alternative pedagogy with different motivations to mainstream education it is unsurprising that progressive educators also conceptualize the learner differently. In contrast to the heavily criticized, but arguably still widely used deficit models in education, progressives operate on an asset-based model in the belief that everybody already has some form of valuable knowledge prior to formal learning. Furthermore, many progressive educators believe learning to be an innate human ability, one that people retain throughout their lives, and which flourishes under voluntary rather than mandatory conditions (Jarvis, 1987; Green et al., 2015). Acknowledging what people *do have* and *can do* rather than what they apparently do not have or cannot do, opens up the possibility of non-hierarchical relationships based on mutuality. This has a direct influence upon the communicative process and crucially forms the basis for any learning that is generated thereafter. This approach, which has been used successfully for some time in adult education and community development in the UK (Mayo and Thompson, 1995), has transformed 'powerless' individuals with very poor self esteem from disadvantaged communities into active citizens who have then gone on to apply their intimate knowledge with that what they have learned to transform their own communities in turn.

Implication for Practice 1

Working in a progressive way means acknowledging that people's attitudes, values and behaviour are shaped by their past and present circumstances. By establishing supportive, non-hierarchical relationships practitioners can learn more about people's lives and the challenges they face. Such insights allow professionals to be more accepting of people and to show more understanding, providing a sound basis for effective, non-judgemental communication.

Such clear illustrations of empowerment have not gone unnoticed by health promotion practitioners who, guided by the values of the Ottawa Charter (WHO, 1986), have increasingly deployed asset-based community development approaches to enable people to take control of their health (South et al., 2013). Central to health promotion then is the theory of empowerment – a set of Freirean ideas about education which have traditionally underpinned both the theory and practice in health promotion. Embedded within empowerment theory is the much needed blueprint for practice that promises to transform 'The Oppressed' into agents for change, agents who can then go on to prepare others to bring about transformations at an organizational or societal level (Allman and Wallis, 1995). Yet despite the promise of empowerment and the rhetoric of policy makers, academics and practitioners, there is ample evidence to suggest that people have not become empowered and taken control of their health. So has empowerment lost its power as Woodall et al. (2012) claim? In light of this critique, it is perhaps timely to reappraise the continuing relevance of Freire's educational ideas to health communication and health promotion, and to consider in detail some of the challenges associated with the empowerment approach.

Paulo Freire: the theory of empowerment and its contribution to health communication

Paulo Freire (1921–1997). A Brazilian educationalist who worked with illiterate adults in Brazil in 1947 where he developed a method of work called *conscientization*. In the 1960s his method received federal government support, facilitating work with over 200,000 adults in every Brazilian state. In 1964 he became Professor of History and Philosophy of Education in the University of Recife but following a coup d'état was imprisoned by the new regime and later forced into exile. From 1969–70 he was Visiting Professor at Harvard University before taking up a post as a special consultant in the Office of Education for the World Council of Churches, Geneva. Freire returned to Brazil in 1979 and till 1985 led the adult literacy project for the Workers' Party, São Paulo. In 1988 Paulo Freire was appointed as São Paulo's Secretary of Education. Key texts: *Pedagogy of the Oppressed* (1972); *Pedagogy of Hope. Reliving Pedagogy of the Oppressed* (1995).

Freire's theory of empowerment

If we agree that the core business of health promotion centres upon transformational activities designed to enable individuals and communities to take control, then Freire's concept of empowerment remains useful to the practitioner. However, the constituent elements of empowerment have significant implications for health communication – which we will consider now.

Dialogue

The key to empowering individuals and communities is the method of its facilitation: dialogue. Dialogue is a form of *group* communication and is the bedrock of all action-oriented learning. Dialogue replaces the need for standardized codified curricula that characterize mainstream education because it begins from the premise that individuals are already knowledgeable. Using people's life experiences (or practical knowledge) forms the basis of communication in Freirean dialogue and the role of the facilitator is one of posing critical questions about those lived experiences to tease out the hidden, constructed nature of social reality – and indeed of knowledge itself.

Dialogue therefore requires the practitioner to have a keen understanding of the socio-economic and political factors that shape (directly and indirectly) people's health and well-being. It also requires a holistic appreciation of health and how the hidden hand of power works to structure inequalities in general and health inequalities in particular – both within and between societies (Pickett and Wilkinson, 2009). Health communication in the form of dialogue is demanding because, besides having an excellent subject knowledge, practitioners need to have the full range of 'wicked competencies' listed by Knight (2007) as the ability to develop supportive relationships; emotional intelligence; group work; listening and assimilation skills; oral communication and an ability to relate to clients as well as being able to self-manage and take things forward. This is indeed a sophisticated skill-set and includes practices usually associated with youth and community work; community development and informal education rather than health promotion. Being 'humble' (Freire, 1972) could also be included as a 'wicked competency' – one which plays a vital role in negotiating entry and acceptance into a group or community, but also in establishing the basis for non-hierarchical relationships and communication.

Implication for Practice 2

Education-as-communication requires practitioners to develop their communication and facilitation skills with an emphasis on the 'wicked competencies'. Practitioners should actively seek to develop these skills and work with other disciplines to provide such opportunities.

Treating people as assets and not as 'passive sensors of given facts' (Bhaskar, 1989: 49–50) is a liberating communication experience that is as inclusive as it is authentic, because it is necessarily predicated upon the discussion of interesting 'real life' issues which encourage genuine engagement. This form of communication is practical and action oriented: it is designed to involve people in the co-production of knowledge so that they might at some point become agents in the world and act on those important existential issues. Thus, dialogue in the Freirean sense is an overtly *political* activity principally designed to foster a critical awareness and develop agency.

Seen in this way, dialogue represents a radical departure from the communication theories prevalent in health promotion, tending as they do to promote the binaries of 'senders' and 'receivers'. These theories advance the notion that health messages are already formed by the practitioner (sender) *prior* to meeting the group or community (receivers) which is highly problematic for practitioners who claim to act in the emancipatory tradition because it presupposes much of what progressives believe *cannot* be known or *should* not be assumed. Only through dialogue, a communication method arising from mutual respect and a concern for one another's welfare, can both practitioners and group members fully come to understand each other and appreciate the impact of complex structural socio-economic and political forces on health.

Despite the increasing sophistication of communication theories (as outlined in the previous chapter), they continue to promote a deficit model of communication that privileges the role of the expert, whose activities primarily centre on 'banking' bits of health information with the 'receivers' rather than fostering a sense of agency and power within an informal learning collective.

Knowledge

The concept that knowledge is socially structured and controlled is one of Freire's most important contributions to education theory because it liberates ordinary men and women from being cast as passive 'empty vessels' to being co-producers of knowledge and potentially very powerful agents of change (Jarvis, 1987). This radically different concept of knowledge contrasts sharply with the positivist concepts that dominate mainstream education today which understand knowledge to be 'fixed'.

> While in education for domestication one cannot speak of a knowable object but only of knowledge which is complete, which the educator possesses and transfers to the educatee, in education for liberation there is no complete knowledge possessed by the educator, but a knowable object which mediates educator and educatee as subjects in the knowing process. (Freire, 1974: 20–1)

Knowledge in empowerment theory is an action-oriented process of collaboration and co-production between participants and practitioners who, through dialogue, make explicit their own individual assumptions about a subject to arrive at a deeper, more critical understanding of a world that is constantly moving and changing (Allman, 1988). This offers a sound theoretical basis for egalitarian relationships and practices which promote democracy through participation, encouraging a flat 'hierarchy' where practitioners learn from participants as well as the more traditional relationship in which the participants learn from practitioners. This is key to understanding the transformational aspects of Freirean empowerment theory which we go into more detail in the final section on *conscientization*.

In terms of health communication, this privileges the personal experiences of the collective over the expert knowledge of the professional. This too is problematic because interpreting knowledge gained from individual experience throws up a diversity of fallible perspectives that have been forged from our gender, race and class positions in society (Archer, 1995). Therefore, it is incumbent upon the health communicator acting in the Freirean tradition to recognize this, and using a theoretical understanding of intersectionality (Gopaldas, 2013) move the group beyond personal identity politics and individualistic causation theories that focus on personal responsibility for 'lifestyle choices' to critically investigate the structural origins of inequality that determine health. This concept of knowledge for action is closely tied to the Aristotelian concept of praxis (2004) which is also a constituent part of Freire's empowerment theory.

Praxis

For Freire, knowledge should ultimately serve a useful purpose and as we outlined earlier in the chapter, the purpose of emancipatory education is to bring about transformations in individuals and society so that all might share in the 'good life' (Aristotle, 2004: 209). The 'good life' is a condition in which all human life may flourish, meaning it is a life in which people move beyond their own individual and exclusive concerns to care for the health and well-being of others generally. Thus, as Smith (1999, 2011) points out, praxis requires an understanding of other people – what the Greeks called *phronesis* – and the ability to 'move between the particular and the general'; or to put it another way, an ability to move from the personal to the political. Praxis, in short, is action-oriented, collective practical wisdom used to bring about positive transformations in the world at an individual, community and societal level.

Necessarily grounded in the Freirean concepts of knowledge and dialogue, praxis in a health promotion setting means that practitioners cannot know *in advance* the particular focus of communication or the means (methods) that might be deployed to realize particular goals. As Bernstein (1983) explains, the end itself only emerges through deliberating about the means appropriate to a *particular* situation. The major implication for the practitioner communicating health, as we have already highlighted above, is that there can be no prior knowledge of the issues that will actually emerge through dialogue and because of this, no ready-made messages. One might argue that given the wealth of detailed information available to the professional today, the practitioner could estimate the kind of issues of concern and thus prepare a suitable health intervention in advance. However, to do this would circumvent the process vital to empowerment itself and so much of that process depends upon the powerful interplay of complex socio-cultural forces (Archer, 2000) that happen to be situated within dynamic 'spatio-temporalities' (Bhaskar, 1998: 603–4).

This essentially locates all players (professional and lay) as subjects of a particular time and place which is why the communicator-as-facilitator should orient their practice to the present. Rooted in the here and now, the concerns of the health communicator-as-facilitator become inextricably linked to the prescient concerns of the group, changing the practitioner's focus from a preoccupation with codified knowledge about health to one that is attentive to the group's physical and emotional needs. As a result, there is greater consideration of the 'learning' environment in which communication takes place and a greater amount of time is spent on the continuous improvement of 'wicked competencies', prompting the practitioner to investigate other progressive theories such as Rogers' work on relationships (1961, 1980); Gardener's theory of multiple intelligences – including emotional intelligence (1983, 1993); Lewin's insights into group work (1948); and Culley and Bond's work on listening skills (2004). Indeed, without a sound knowledge of educational theory and the insights it provides about progressive praxis, it is difficult to imagine how the professional health promoter might structure communication-as-empowerment.

Conscientization

At the heart of empowerment theory is *conscientization* which Freire describes as 'learning to perceive social, political, and economic contradictions, and to take action against the oppressive elements of reality' (1972:16, footnote). Taylor calls this process 'developing consciousness' (1993:52) and he distinguishes it from other forms of awareness-raising by its *transformative* powers which Allman and Wallis refer to as the ability to 'prepare people, who will go on to prepare others, to transform their social relations at all levels' (1995:19). In this emancipatory process Freire communicates his beliefs about the potential for all human beings – even the powerless and the oppressed – to learn, and, specifically through dialogue and praxis arrive at a critical view of reality which, according to Archer (1995, 2000), is necessary for the formation of human agency. Herein lies the rub, because the potential for agency only exists if men and women first discover *for themselves* the constructed nature of social reality (and therefore the constructed nature of inequality and oppression also). As Horton explains, true learning can only ever result from a process of internalizing knowledge gained through experience and reflected upon by analysis and a commitment to action (Horton, cited in Jarvis, 1987).

This is not to say that the health communicator-as-facilitator does not play an important role in structuring such discoveries, but it is of crucial importance to the process of acquiring agency that group members do their *own* learning and are encouraged to draw their own conclusions from experience. Once the practitioner understands and accepts this, and that there can be no place for information or knowledge transfer when educating for empowerment, their concept of what it means to be a professional 'delivering' health communication is forever changed – as they too become transformed by the process of *conscientization*.

In purposefully creating opportunities for dialogue and nurturing every possibility to develop agency, the role of the health communicator working in the Freirean tradition becomes overtly political – and because of this 'dangerous' (Green et al., 2015: 366). Conscientization is dangerous because it is a form of action-oriented education that intentionally sets out to challenge the hegemonic powers of the Establishment, which according to Bourdieu and Passeron,

> [R]eproduce the dominant culture, contributing thereby to the reproduction of the structure of power relationships with a social formation in which the dominant system of education tends to secure a monopoly of legitimate symbolic violence. (Bourdieu and Passeron, 1990: 6)

For healthcare professionals working within a welfare state *conscientization* represents a direct challenge to state authority and as such cannot realistically expect any support from it (Brookfield, 1987). This is because *conscientization* essentially means taking action against the people, policies and structures that give rise to such gross health inequalities. Seen in this way, we come to understand why Freirean education is perceived as a potential threat to the state, particularly when its collectivist values oppose the current and dominant neoliberal individualistic policies that promote free market expansion in public services; transforming what was once regarded as an essential public good into a private luxury (Kurlich, 1992, cited in Heaney, 1996). The implications of this should be of concern to those who believe that a publicly funded, comprehensive and universal National Health Service is not only necessary for a healthy society, but a more equal society and the essential foundation of social and economic progress.

Implication for Practice 3
Practitioners should continually develop their experience and knowledge *vis-à-vis* health inequalities to acquire a sound practical wisdom of the issues. A useful way to do this is to receive regular communication feeds from reputable sources and to become involved in local, regional and national networks that are working to combat the effects of, and the reduction of health inequalities.

Besides being 'dangerous', emancipatory practices associated with *conscientization* are also 'difficult' because of the sophisticated skill-set that is required of the practitioner as highlighted earlier. Green et al. (2015) believe that this difficulty has increasingly led practitioners to adapt Freirean concepts and adopt 'pseudo-Freirean' practices (Kidd and Kumar, 1981) which, while using the rhetoric of empowerment, do not challenge the status quo. As a result, Freire's ideas have, over time, become emasculated and what once signalled a powerful key concept in health promotion has, according to Woodall et al. (2012), become little more than 'a buzzword'. However, it is not only health promoters who have struggled to put empowerment theory into practice: radical adult educators have too, and since the mid 1990s been on the receiving end of an attack which has completely restructured some of the most important ideological sites for the development and reproduction of empowerment theory in the UK. The story of Community Education in Scotland serves as a sobering example of what happens when the values of the market are applied to public higher education and introduce into it an audit culture where professional work is evaluated to a positivist 'uniform metric' (Corbett, 2008). For details, see Shaw and Crowther (1995).

This metric ultimately re-frames what is of value, squeezing out the possibility for alternative pedagogies to exist and it is here, in the ideological restructuring of public services, that the real dangers and difficulties to transformational praxis lie; for once the performative forces of commodification and marketization take hold (Bourdieu and Passeron, 1990), they proliferate, increasing content-based forms of education that reinforce market values, redefining the notion of 'success'. According to Sears these developments represent 'an active policy of extending market discipline . . . [in which] the decommodified spaces of education are being eroded as part of the elimination of any spaces outside market relations' (2003: 18 ff).

Since the early 1990s similar forces have also been at work within the NHS in the UK, extending and escalating the market discipline to commodify (and marketize) products and services through the introduction of Private Finance Initiatives (PFI) and competitive tendering through clinical commissioning. These developments have forced a business agenda upon the NHS and fostered a managerial culture that is at pains to illustrate value for money within the term of a general election. Within local authority public health departments where health promotion activities are now situated, this results in 'downstream' health promotion interventions that promise tangible outcomes – often captured by changes in behaviour. In this climate, there is little room for empowerment theory because the values and practices associated with it do not align with current conceptualizations of what public health is and what health promoters ought to do. Health promotion in the Freirean tradition would in any case resist the ubiquitous toolkit approach and most likely fail the positivist quality assurance frameworks currently in operation.

Yet, despite the obstructive policies which presently shape professional practice it is vital that health promoters safeguard the principles and practices of empowerment because it is effective in tackling inequality, which according to Shiller (Shiller, 2013, cited in Dorling, 2015), is the most important problem we face today. For these reasons practitioners should not abandon their social justice commitments, but perhaps in light of the very real 'dangers and difficulties' associated with empowerment in the workplace they should consider some worthy alternatives. John Dewey's progressive theory of educative experience and Martin Buber's relational theory of education offer radical practitioners just that, and while not *overtly* political, support much of what health promoters have come to value in Freirean empowerment theory. Originating in the early part of the twentieth century, these ideas still have much to offer practitioners today – especially those who work informally with people from disadvantaged communities because they reveal what is most important in the educative process, and in doing so, provide an authentic account of 'what works'.

John Dewey: the importance of experience and democracy in education

John Dewey (1859–1952). An American philosopher and educator; pioneer in functional psychology; founder of Pragmatism and leader of the Progressive Movement (US). From 1884 he taught philosophy and psychology at the University of Michigan. From 1894–1904 he

> ### Implication for Practice 4
>
> Effective health communication or health messages cannot be prepared in advance without compromising the principles of empowerment in action. This is an obvious truism, because in anticipating what might emerge from a group the practitioner focuses on their own professional knowledge (and values) rather than on relationship-building. Building relationships can be challenging and this part of the work is often difficult to evidence 'as work' so it is useful to think about how this underpins the health promotion intervention.

developed an experimental progressive pedagogy at the University of Chicago before joining Columbia University, New York, where he spent most of his career. Key texts: *Democracy in Education* (1916); *How We Think. A restatement of the relation of reflective thinking to the educative process* (1933); *Experience and Education* (1938).

Dewey's Philosophy of Education Based on Experience

Although Dewey's theory situates him firmly within the modern progressive movement in education, his ideas about the purpose of education date back to Greek Antiquity, and Aristotle in particular. For like Aristotle Dewey believed education should ultimately serve a civic function and in his words, prepare people, 'for future responsibilities and success in life' (Dewey, 1997:18). Dewey's ideas also draw upon the Aristotelian concept of *phronesis* (practical wisdom) and he encourages the use of knowledge gained through personal experience to enhance participation in the learning process. In all this Dewey emphasizes the facilitator's ability to nurture positive relationships – another defining characteristic of transformational learning theory shared by ancient and modern progressive educators. For these reasons we should consider Dewey's philosophy of education based on experience to evaluate whether its key principles of continuity, quality and democracy have a potential application to health communication in health promotion theory and praxis.

Principle 1: The Continuity of Experience

Dewey advocates the use of personal experience as the basis for learning as it generates a rich, informally derived curriculum that is of genuine interest to learners, creating a motivation for learning. This engenders a democratic arrangement of relationships that reposition the professional from, 'the position of boss or dictator to take on the role of a facilitator of group activities' (Dewey, 1997: 59). This resonates with both Freire's conceptualization of knowledge and Johnson's notion of 'really useful knowledge' and the role of the facilitator, requiring in each case a high level of skill in the 'wicked competencies' as well as a, 'well-thought-out philosophy of the social factors that operate in the constitution of experience' (Dewey, 1997: 21).

That said, not all experiences are educative in Dewey's opinion: indeed some can be mis-educative in that they close down (or fail to offer up in the first place) the future possibility of an authentic, challenging learning experience and a valuable opportunity for personal growth. For Dewey, educative experiences are those which are: (a) democratic, (b) engaging, (c) challenging (rather than merely enjoyable) and (d) *linked,* giving the learner a sense of continuity in learning – or as Dewey puts it, an *'experiential continuum'* (1997:33). This continuum, structured by the facilitator using personal contributions, enables the learner to build their knowledge cumulatively over time, allowing them also to acquire good habits for learning and thereby avoid becoming 'scatter-brained' (ibid, 26). Central to this process is Dewey's notion of *collateral learning* which he believed should be strengthened to foster a *desire* for learning (1997: 48). Thus, the primary role of the educator/facilitator is to nurture the development of positive attitudes towards learning and in doing so, effectively shift the attention from what is to be learned, i.e. content (knowledge) to focus instead upon the mindset of the learner and to bring about change therein.

This clearly departs from traditional educational theory which privileges content over process, but it is also a departure from many progressive theories too. This is evident *vis-à-vis* Freire's theory of empowerment and Johnson's concept of 'really useful knowledge' because even though both perspectives advance the primacy of process they still retain a central focus on knowledge – socially constructed knowledge perhaps, but knowledge nonetheless. In relocating the focus to the attitudinal rather than the cognitive or indeed the affective domains of learning, Dewey has authored a theory of progressive education that is ideally suited to the twenty-first century: a time in which knowledge (and indeed those who interpret knowledge) has arguably lost some of its value. The revolution in information technology and global communications has altered every aspect of modern life, fundamentally changing our habits and relationship with information, knowledge and communication. These advances have, within a generation, elevated the importance of media in our personal and professional lives, making information available to all within reach of a personal computer or smartphone. But is being information-rich the same as being knowledgeable? Green et al. contend that the, 'mere transmission of information is not the same as the relatively permanent change in knowledge, disposition or capability which is central to . . . learning' (2015: 299). So while information is almost certainly a necessary prerequisite for learning, it does not adequately describe the complex dynamic communication processes associated with acquiring knowledge. For that, a theory of education is needed that equips people with the skills to learn as well as a positive attitude to learning, enabling them to value knowledge for themselves throughout the lifecourse.

Principle 2: The Quality of Educational Experience

Dewey's concern for people to develop a positive mental attitude towards learning and to acquire good learning habits demands a person-centred approach – which brings us onto the second key principle of Dewey's theory: the quality of the educational experience. According to Dewey (1997), the interaction between the facilitator and the learners is inseparable from the situation itself and therefore it is imperative that the facilitator be attentive to this and the needs of the learners present. Usefully Dewey reminds us that professional practice should be grounded in the present for 'we live at the time we live and not at some other' (1997: 49). This requires the facilitator to set up a positive learning environment that enables interaction and so careful consideration in the planning and execution is necessary. To do this effectively, the facilitator must know the needs of the learners and this can only be known if time is taken to develop such relationships (Dewey, 1997). No standard approach can be adopted, which runs counter to current wisdom in public health and health promotion where there is an array of standardized materials and 'readymade' toolkits available for the practitioner to use (www.networks.nhs.uk). Dewey would have been critical of such approaches, impressing upon practitioners that in order to interest and engage people in an active knowledge-making process they 'cannot start with knowledge already organized and proceed to ladle it out in doses' (1997: 82).

Attempts to short-circuit this process for reasons of time and efficiency result in a mis-educative experience as practitioners-as-facilitators fail to engage learners meaningfully. In adhering to the constituent features that inform the quality of educational experience (i.e. interaction and situation) Dewey suggests facilitators devote their attentions to the students before them and to negotiate with them democratically those educative experiences which have the potential to fulfil the principle of the *experiential continuum*. These two principles essentially give us the *what* and *how* of learning in Dewey's theory; the third principle gives us the reason *why*, to which we now turn.

Principle 3: Democracy in Education and Education for Democracy

At the heart of Dewey's educational theory is a concern to preserve the humanistic values of democratic societies which, if not actively renewed through educative means, he feared would return even the most civilized of groups to 'barbarism and savagery' (Dewey, 2008: 4). Practising democracy *educatively* means communicating authentically with 'fullness and accuracy' giving participants an enlarged, enlightened and changed experience (Dewey, 2008: 6). Thus, Dewey believed the experience of an alternative pedagogy was in itself transformational, triggering a fundamental change in people and modifying their attitudes beyond the confines of the immediate learning environment to affect the quality of subsequent experiences (Dewey, 1997). Therein lies the value of transformational learning because, unlike cognitive forms of learning, the affective nature of democratic communication challenges our basic sensitivities, providing a useful, alternative set of relations which help us respond to all the conditions we meet in life.

The linchpin of Dewey's philosophy is *communication*, because it is in communication that society *exists*; it is how the aims, beliefs, aspirations and knowledge which constitute democratic society are transmitted. Democratic society can only be achieved (and maintained) through communication, which in turn ensures participation; and through participation we have the means to understand one another and form a consensus. The ability to reach a consensus is essential if people are to share a 'common life' (Dewey, 2008: 9), 'in which all individuals have an opportunity to contribute something, and in which the activities in which all participate are the chief carrier of control' (Dewey, 1997: 56). However, it is clear from Dewey's definition that many individuals, despite sharing similar social or economic circumstances, do not share in a common life. Instead, they exist upon a 'machine like plane' and act instrumentally to get the outcomes they desire. This, for Dewey, results in inauthentic communication (2008: 5). True communication requires individuals to give much more of themselves, and for further insight as to how this might be achieved we look to Buber's ideas about the nature of dialogue.

Martin Buber: developing true dialogue and mutuality in communication

Martin Buber (1878–1965) Jewish theologian and philosopher. Student of philosophy, art history, German studies and psychology at the University of Vienna. Editor of the Zionist weekly: *Die Welt* (The World); founder and editor of *Der Jude* (The Jew) in which he advocated the formation of a Jewish-Arab state in Palestine. Honorary professor at the University of Frankfurt (1930); Head of the Jewish Adult Education College in Frankfurt-am-Main (1933); Director of the Jewish Adult Education College in Frankfurt-am-Main in 1934. Forced to emigrate to Palestine in 1938. From 1938–51 he was professor of the Hebrew University of Jerusalem; the first president of the Israeli Academy of Sciences and Art and founder of the Teachers Training College for Adult Education in Jerusalem. Key texts: *I and Thou* (1958); *Paths in Utopia* (1946); *Between* Man *and Man* (1947).

Buber's definition of dialogue necessitates a 'turning towards the other' (Buber, 2004: 25) which he considered a vital precursor to two indispensable forms of true human life: (a) sharing in an undertaking and (b) entering into mutuality' (Buber, 2004: 103). This form of communication privileges the attitude of students above cognitive ability because as Buber declares, 'there are no gifted and ungifted here, only those who give themselves and those who withhold themselves' (2004: 40). For Buber, the process of sharing oneself is educative and so, in common with both Dewey and Freire, he advances a theory of educative practice that is *relational* rather than fixed on a set curriculum. Buber describes the practice of opening up oneself to the other as 'communion' (2004: 108) which he believed developed when people experience a sense of freedom in learning. This contrasts with compulsion in education which gives rise to humiliation and rebelliousness. Thus, the role of the facilitator in dialogical learning is to create the freedom for people to learn and to foster trusting, inclusive relationships that allow for 'communion' to take place.

According to Buber, the quality of the relationship between persons (between the practitioner and lay person) is characterized by the element of inclusion which he terms 'the dialogical relation' (2004: 115). Failure to be inclusive and involve others in a true dialogue runs the risk of the facilitator being drawn into a position of authority where they arbitrarily choose a curriculum that is primarily of concern to them, and not a negotiated curriculum that is drawn from the student's own reality. As with Dewey's principle of quality which suggests facilitators focus primarily on the situation and inter-action, Buber asks facilitators to consider the student experience for,

> The man whose calling it is to influence the being of persons . . . must experience this action of his (however much it may have assumed the form of non-action) ever anew from the other side. (Buber, 2004: 118)

If inclusion forms an essential part of Buberian dialogue so too does the element of friendship which, in line with ancient and modern progressive educational traditions, demands that facilitators show a genuine concern for the person, 'both in the actuality in which he lives before you now and in his possibilities, what he can become' (Buber, 2004: 123). It is within this relationship of mutuality, founded upon inclusivity and friendship that the facilitator may come to mould an individual's character. Buber acknowledges that character is influ-enced by a number of complex opposing and intersecting influences, but among this infinity of forces the facilitator is unique because of the *active* desire to shape a person's character by the selection of what is *right* and what *should be* (Buber, 2004: 123). However, Buber con-tends that to shape another's character outside 'the dialogical relation' is unethical – but not once confidence has been won because when this happens there exists a positive, mutual relationship where genuine communication begins – and it is at this point that the 'student' begins to *ask*. Confidence is won not by the endeavour to win it, but by the facilitator's 'direct and ingenious participation' in the lives of those she or he works with (Buber, 2004: 127). That said, Buber reminds us that even when one enjoys the confidence of those s/he seeks, the facilitator cannot always expect agreement; however, if handled well, conflict can be used educatively – this is the acid test for the educator!

Dewey, Buber and Freire diverge in their intent, but their edu-cational theories have much in common: the primacy of experience and communication in the educative process; a commitment to non-hierarchical and inclusive relationships and the desire to enter into authentic, dynamic dialogue with others that is purposefully transformational. Education-as-communication is used to enlighten and develop an informed, active citizenry who, once transformed by their educative experience, go on to transform others and the world to create a more tolerable society – one that is fairer, more equal and just.

Summary of key points

This chapter has given a critical overview of transformative education and appraised its contribution to health communication in promoting health. Specifically it has:

- described the key features of progressive educational theory in relation to health communication praxis in health promotion
- evaluated the continuing relevance of Freire's empowerment theory to health promotion and examined the difficulties and dangers associated with this approach
- explored the educational ideas of Buber and Dewey to provide a complementary alternative to Freirean empowerment theory in health communication and health promotion
- considered the implications for health communication and for professional practitioners in health promotion

Reflection 1 – How should radical practitioners prepare for educative encounters if they do not rely on toolkits and ready-made materials?

Reflection 2 – Can the radical health promoter deploy a form of emancipatory praxis that can satisfy outcomes-based quality assurance frameworks for health?

Reflection 3 – What are the personal and professional challenges that attend Buber's interpretation of dialogue?

Reflection 4 – How does the concept of radical health communication praxis challenge our understanding of the 'expert' and professional practice?

Further reading

Jarvis, P. (ed.) (1987) *Twentieth-Century Thinkers in Adult Education.* London and New York: Routledge. This is an examination of the work of seventeen major thinkers in the field of adult and continuing education, showing how each has made a significant contribution to the field.
Jeffs, T. and Smith, M. K. (1999) *Informal Education. Conversation, Democracy and Learning.* 2nd edn. Ticknall: Education Now Books. This

book explores how informal educators encourage conversation, democracy and learning.

Thompson, J. (1993) Learning, liberation and maturity. An open letter to Whoever's Left. *Adults Learning*, 4 (9), 244. This open letter reflects upon the increasing marketization in education and the loss of 'really useful knowledge' and consciousness-raising as part of the adult education experience.

4

Psychological Theory

Key aims

- To give a brief overview of several 'classic' theories of behaviour change
- To examine key concepts in psychological theory such as the influence of others, self-esteem and notions of control
- To present a generic critique of behaviour change theory originating in psychology
- To consider the importance of context and meaning for health behaviour and the implications for health communication
- To introduce alternative approaches to understanding health behaviour

Introduction

This chapter will draw on theories of behaviour change from the discipline of psychology. It will outline the key theoretical approaches to understanding the process of behaviour change and consider what the evidence is to support these. It will draw on international research to examine the complexities of human behaviour and describe the key approaches which are taken. Key theories will be briefly outlined, and then critiqued. These will include the 'classic' major theories in this field such as the Health Belief Model, the Theory of Reasoned Action and the Theory of Planned Behaviour, the Trans-Theoretical Model and Protection Motivation Theory. The chapter will then introduce and critique other innovations in behaviour change theory such as Social Psychological Theory concerned with the influence of others, the notion of self-esteem and perceptions of control and two further specific theories – the Behavioural Ecological Model and the Theory of Triadic Influence. Throughout this chapter relevant research findings will be drawn upon to illustrate key points and enhance the discussion, bringing theoretical features to life.

Psychology is a key discipline in health communication and health promotion. Understanding how people think, feel and behave is extremely important in terms of health and efforts to maximize health gain. We can turn to psychology to develop this understanding. Psychology, as a discipline, is huge, so for the purposes of this chapter it is only possible to give relatively brief mention of some of the myriad of theories that attempt to describe and explain human behaviour. We have chosen to start with some of the classic, relatively well-known theories that, rightly or wrongly, dominate the academic literature. We only briefly present these since they are well-rehearsed within the wider literature.

This chapter sets out to trouble received wisdom about health behaviour and the focus on individual behaviour change as the primary means to health gain in a neoliberal climate dominated by Western values (as defined in Chapter 1). It will critique the way that received wisdom is uncritically accepted and reproduced in non-Western contexts where 'more Westernized lifestyles' are changing epidemiologic patterns of disease; for example, the rise of chronic so-called 'lifestyle' diseases in emerging middle-classes in Zambia (Rudatsikira et al., 2012).

We might reasonably argue that the ultimate aim of *all* health promotion and communication efforts is to change behaviour, whether it is through creating supportive environments or via the vehicle of healthy public policy. In fact, it is difficult to think of an example which refutes this. Nevertheless this chapter will focus on psychological theory as applied to health communication and health promotion.

'Classic' theories of health behaviour and behaviour change

A number of theories about behaviour and behaviour change abound within academic literature. For more in-depth information readers are encouraged to engage with the suggested further reading at the end of this chapter. Here we focus on the theories that are most prevalent.

Health belief model (HBM)

The health belief model was developed as an attempt to explain why people do not take up preventative and/or protective health behaviours (Salazar et al., 2013). The HBM proposes that an individual is more likely to take action to take up behaviours dependent on a range of different *beliefs*. These include beliefs about susceptibility to a condition, the severity of a condition and the benefits/costs of making a change. In addition, a set of individual demographic variables (age, gender, socio-economic status) are considered to influence beliefs, as can different 'cues to action' such as symptoms of ill-health or health communication efforts. Self-efficacy is a further variable relating to the belief in one's ability to carry out a specific action or to change behaviour. All these variables combined lead to 'the likelihood of taking action'. A great deal of research has used the HBM to try to understand and determine behaviour, not just protective behaviour but health behaviours more generally (Hayden, 2014). There has, however, been no standard approach to this and studies have applied the constructs within the HBM in different ways (Rodham, 2010). It is therefore difficult to compare findings in a meaningful way.

Nevertheless, the literature reports numerous studies within different global contexts. The HBM has been used to try to explain adherence to self-care or health-promoting behaviours (Wai Sze Lo et al., 2015 – Hong Kong; Abolfotouh et al., 2015 – Kingdom of Saudi Arabia); to evaluate interventions, for example, in a school injury prevention programme (Cao et al., 2014 – China); to design interventions aimed at, for example, reducing alcohol use (El-Rahman et al., 2014 – Egypt) and to increase physical activity in women at risk of hypertension (Hoseini et al., 2014 – Iran). Evidently, despite the criticisms levelled at it, the Health Belief Model is still widely in use. In a meta-analysis by Carpenter (2010) the two variables with highest predictive value were benefits and barriers but this highlighted limitations within the model. Interestingly there is a relative dearth of systematic meta-analytic research on the HBM.

The theories of reasoned action and planned behaviour (TRA and TPB)

The theory of reasoned action suggests that behavioural intention is directly linked to behaviour and can be predicted by two constructs:

the *attitude towards the behaviour* which refers to how someone feels about engaging in a particular behaviour; and *subjective norm* which refers to what the individual thinks their significant others will think about them behaving differently. The theory of planned behaviour (Ajzen, 1988) includes a third construct, *perceived behavioural control*. This refers to the extent to which the individual believes they are capable of taking up the new behaviour (Crosby et al., 2013a). It is viewed, by some, as similar to the concept of self-efficacy. Attention has been given to the so-called *intention-behaviour gap* (Rodham, 2010). The focus on behavioural intention at the expense of actual behaviour has been criticized and the relationship shown to be weak (Rhodes and Dickau, 2012) although it is acknowledged that we are more likely to do something if we have an intention to do so (Hayden, 2014).

In a systematic review on dietary behaviour interventions for adolescents and young adults Hackman and Knowlden (2014) concluded that further research was needed to 'identify the optimal TPB and TRA modalities to modify dietary behaviours' (p. 101). This is not peculiar to TPB and TRA, however. A systematic review and meta-analysis of social cognitive theories and physical activity behaviour in adolescents found inconsistent evidence and also concluded that further research was needed because the majority of variance remained unexplained (Plotnikoff et al., 2013). A cursory glance at the literature shows limitations in the utility of the TPB. The main focus is on the predictive validity of the different constructs in terms of whether each leads to an increased intention to perform a specific behaviour. The lack of a consistent approach means that several meta-analyses and systematic reviews have been generally inconclusive. For example, a meta-analysis found that TPB explains only a fifth of the variance in behaviour and less than half of the variation in behavioural intention (McEachan et al., 2011). Results also vary according to the type of behaviour. It seems that the theory is more useful in predicting certain types of behaviour such as physical activity and dietary practices. A further challenge is that the TPB is often used in combination with other models such as the HBM (Tyson et al., 2014). Given these limitations Sniehotta et al. (2014: 4) suggest that the TPB is 'retired' arguing that it is 'no longer a plausible theory of behaviour or behaviour change'. Disappointingly, however, they advocate a range of individualized, deductive, hypothetical approaches to understanding behaviour instead.

Implication for Practice 1
When planning health communication interventions it is important to take people's beliefs into account and to recognize the role that culture, social norms and context play in the creation of these. We need to begin with a very good understanding of where people are and take into account lay perspectives. Involving people (primary stakeholders) at the planning stage is therefore absolutely crucial to success.

Trans-theoretical model (TTM)

The TTM (Prochaska and DiClemente, 1984) is a stage theory that describes the stages which people may go through in changing behaviour. The TTM has been used to change behaviour in a wide range of different issues including the adoption of healthier practices and the cessation of unhealthy ones (DiClemente et al., 2013). The TTM outlines five stages through which individuals move sequentially towards permanent behaviour change. These are pre-contemplation, contemplation, preparation, action and maintenance. A sixth stage, termination, is also included. In each stage people show different levels of willingness to change. The purpose of health communication efforts is to move people on through the different stages. Methods may be tailored according to where a person is in the cycle. The model has been adopted as a diagnostic tool for establishing readiness to change on the assumption that people can be categorized into the different stages (DiClemente et al., 2013). Alongside the defined stages of change Prochaska and DiClemente (1984) outline ten processes of change – consciousness raising, dramatic relief, self-re-evaluation, self-liberation, helping relationships, counter-conditioning, contingency management, stimulus control and social liberation. These are the drivers that promote change. Additionally the model includes two other major constructs – self-efficacy and decisional balance. Decisional balance refers to the process of cost/benefit analysis that characterizes value-expectancy theories.

A 2001 meta-analysis concluded that studies using the TTM needed a standardized and reliable means of measurement (Marshall and Biddle, 2001). So far this has not happened. Nevertheless, there appears to be substantial empirical research that supports the use of TTM-tailored approaches in a number of public health areas such as increasing physical activity (Blaney et al., 2012). Results from other studies seem to suggest that the constructs within the TTM have different levels of utility depending on the issue. For example, a study which evaluated the usefulness of the TTM as a basis for interventions to increase fruit and vegetable consumption concluded that the processes of change predicted the people who successfully moved on from pre-contemplation but not those in the preparation stage (Horwath et al., 2013).

Protection motivation theory (PMT)

PMT explains the effect of fear and threat in health communication efforts. Fear appeals are often used to promote health, the premise being that people will seek to avoid perceived threats. PMT posits that, when faced with a threat, people will respond in one of two ways – in an *adaptive* way, where they react positively and avoid the threat, or in a *maladaptive* way, where they will react negatively and ignore the threat. These two outputs result from two appraisal processes. Firstly, *threat appraisal*, in which the person evaluates the seriousness of the threat and the likelihood/severity of a negative outcome, and secondly, *coping appraisal*, in which the person assesses their ability to behave in a way that avoids the threat; this is also referred to as 'efficacy response' (Salazar et al., 2013).

PMT can be used as a theoretical foundation for health communication efforts. For example, in a study in Iran, the theory was used to underpin a health education programme designed to promote behaviours that prevent malaria (Ghahremani et al., 2013). The study concluded that this was a highly effective approach. More often, however, the constructs of the theory are used to predict behavioural intention. Xiao et al. (2014) examined protective behaviours for schistosomiasis infection in China and not all of the constructs within the PMT were significantly associated with behavioural intention. Indeed, results varied across studies for a number of reasons such as definitional inconsistencies.

The influence of others

Social psychology offers us insights which can aid appreciation of human behaviour such as the norms and values that might be specific to certain social or cultural groups. Undoubtedly our shared beliefs and attitudes influence the behavioural choices that we make. This might be for the benefit of our health or to its detriment. Social influence can be considered in a number of different ways. Our friends, our family and wider societal expectations and norms all influence our behaviour. As Manning (2009) argues, there is a substantial body of evidence, in social psychology and beyond, which demonstrates that we conform to the behaviours and judgements of other people. A study in South-East Asia by Sychareun et al. (2013) examined factors affecting premarital heterosexual activity and found that parental expectations and peer influence were predictors of behaviour. A Portuguese study found similar patterns around physical activity in young people (Silva et al., 2014).

A study in Cape Town, South Africa determined that peer pressure was the strongest predictor of substance use (Hendricks et al., 2015). Peer influence appears to be significant in risk-taking behaviour. Young people are more likely to engage in this when in the company of people they consider to be friends (Varela and Pritchard, 2014). An Italian study found that unhealthy behaviours were related to peer-group but also to school environment (Lazzeri et al., 2014). Findings such as these have implications for health communication. Research tends to focus on the detrimental effects of peer influence, particularly in young people and adolescents; however, social influence can also promote healthier behaviour. We have to consider the concept of individual agency here and perhaps question our capacity for agency within a social context. Fitting in with other people's expectations creates social currency; however, in order to do so we may not always behave in ways that reflect the authentic self.

The importance of self-esteem

Self-esteem is an important psychological concept in health behaviours. A Turkish study on self-esteem and health-risk behaviours in late adolescence found that self-esteem was negatively associated with alcohol and illicit drug-use (Kavas, 2009) and a study in Nigeria found that self-esteem was a predictor of adolescents' risky sexual behaviour (Sylvester, 2014). Conversely a study in South Korea (Yeun et al., 2013) concluded that self-esteem does not affect health promotion behaviour in middle-aged Koreans but that self-efficacy does. These examples are fairly typical of mixed results in the wider literature such that it is hard to have firm, definite conclusions. It is also difficult to determine whether higher levels of self-esteem and self-efficacy produce healthier behaviours or vice versa. Higher levels of self-esteem tend to correlate with better mental health as demonstrated by a study which examined physical activity, self-esteem and mental health in ethnic minority students in Chinese colleges (Li et al., 2014). A meta-analysis on self-affirmation concluded that it influences health messages' effect on health intentions and impacts on behaviour (Sweeney and Moyer, 2015). However, the authors also found that, in many of the studies they reviewed, behaviour change was not predicted by intention. Despite the widespread linear assumption underpinning much behaviour change theory, intentions do not always lead to actual behaviour. We have known this for some time yet we seem to persist in the same approaches to research, relying on the same theories!

Implication for Practice 2

Self-esteem is an important concept in promoting healthier behaviours and is known to be central to well-being. Health communication efforts therefore should aim to increase self-esteem in some way. Interventions could include different methods and mechanisms to achieve this such as those that promote self-confidence and mastery.

The concept of control

Control, or perceptions of control, is often linked to behaviour and behaviour change. Behaviour change theory typically constructs the individual as agent and as in control of their behaviour. This assumption has underpinned the neoliberal public health agendas of many Western countries in the past few decades. Neoliberal ideology emphasizes personal freedom and individual control (Brannen and Nilsen, 2005). Control and choice are constructed as freely available to the neoliberal subject (Stuart and Donaghue, 2012). However, the concept of personal control is troublesome and, we would argue, it needs to be scrutinized more closely. For example, the simplistic assumption that lack of control leads to obesity ignores the mitigating effect of living in an obesogenic environment such that self-control becomes a measure of a person's worth (Helén and Jauho, 2003). Tackling an obesogenic environment would mean, for example, acknowledging the role that environmental factors play by addressing the availability of fast foods, lack of safe urban green spaces and the accessible pricing of healthier foods rather than focusing on individuals' diets (Jones et al., 2007).

A generic critique of theories of behaviour change

As argued by Kar et al. (2001a) the theories used in health communication are predicated on research carried out with homogenous populations (white, middle-class, able bodied). Feminist psychologists have long pointed out the historical gender bias in psychological research. The lack of cultural and contextual nuance is also problematic. For example, Sychareun et al. (2013) note the proliferation of research on young people's sexual behaviour in industrialized nations or 'developed' contexts and the lack of it in lower-income countries. In view of such critiques we need to come to any theoretical claims with regard to knowledge about behaviour change with an open and enquiring mind. We need to be conscious of where, and how, that knowledge was brought into being and who is purported to 'own' it.

Writers such as Mielewczyk and Willig (2007) and Robertson and Williams (2010) argue for a move away from an individualistic focus on specific behaviours which characterizes the sociocognitive approaches seen to dominate mainstream health psychology (Stainton-Rogers, 2011). As Zinn (2005) asserts, while expert understanding might link behaviour directly to health, due to the influence of social and cultural factors, lay understandings often do not. The linear assumption that better education or increased awareness leads to behaviour change is inherently problematic (Thompson and Kumar, 2011).

Mielewczyk and Willig (2007) highlight the increasing use, in recent years, of social cognition models (SCMs) in examining health behaviours. They critique these in detail noting theoretical, methodological and performance-based weaknesses. They point to the lack of empirical support for the predictive value of SCMs. However, Mielewczyk and Willig's (2007) paper focuses almost exclusively on critiquing the Theory of Planned Behaviour. SCMs suggest that people are rational actors (Alaszewski, 2005) who carefully consider the potential outcomes of any actions before carrying them out (Salazar et al., 2013). This assumption is problematic and, as such, Alaszewski (2005) argues that risk communication based on assumptions of the rational actor have little effect. Miller (2005) contends that behaviours which might be viewed as irrational might be seen as rational when considered within a specific cultural context, for example, taking part in adrenaline sports. In addition, as Denscombe (2010: 425) argues, 'health-related behaviour is not always rational'.

There are a number of general critiques of theories of behaviour change. Firstly, the focus on factors influencing individual behaviour is at the expense of wider social, political and environmental determinants of health and promotes individual responsibility for health (Airhihenbuwa and Obregon, 2000). While socio-cognitive approaches do acknowledge the role of social context to an extent the reductionist emphasis on the individual (Bunton et al., 2000) tends to 'objectify' human experience and is contrary to a more holistic approach (Green et al., 2015). Theory tends to neglect the role of past behaviour and habit (Upton and Thirlaway, 2014), and of emotion/affect (Lawton et al., 2009). There is a lack of consideration of cultural context and cross-cultural applicability (Lin et al., 2005; Soto Mas et al., 2000). Theory is also criticized for over-simplifying behaviour and behaviour change (Abraham and Sheeran, 2005).

Research using SCMs also raises challenges including problems defining individual constructs (Bunton et al., 2000) which are not standardized across different studies (Connor and Norman, 2015); limited predictive utility (Abraham and Sheeran, 2005); and a weak relationship between intention and behaviour (Stephens, 2008). Flynn et al. (2001) criticize the reliance on mismatched samples. There is often a patriarchal Western bias as the models have been developed in specific contexts. In addition, much of the research relies on self-report measures (Brener et al., 2003). Finally, SCMs do not consider political and economic factors (Hubley and Copeman with Woodall, 2013).

Mielewczyk and Willig (2007) argue that a new approach to research is required which acknowledges the complexity of health behaviours. This echoes a call from Eakin et al. (1996) more than a decade earlier who argued that a critical social science perspective was crucial. Mielewczyk and Willig (2007) contend that one of the major difficulties is the very fact that 'health behaviours' as such do not exist. They acknowledge the term 'health-related behaviours' but their emphasis is on *social context* and the *meaning* that certain types of behaviours may have. They urge that 'health behaviour' is reconceptualized and examined in relation to wider social practices necessitating a more critical perspective. The largely acontextual approaches to exploring health behaviours within mainstream health psychology have also been criticized (see Hepworth, 2004). For example, Chamberlain (2004) questions the focus on eating as a health behaviour and suggests that eating is more about social practices within social contexts arguing that little attention has been paid to the *meaning* that dietary choices and food might have within wider contexts.

Several SCMs include the variable or construct 'risk perception' or 'threat', linking this (to a greater or lesser extent) to intention to behave in a certain way (Gillies and Willig, 1997). This has been criticized on methodological and epistemological grounds. The individualistic focus of these models (which interestingly have appeared in the literature within a similar time-frame to that within which neoliberal economics and politics have gained ground – i.e. from the 1980s onwards) has been called into question by those adopting more critical stances. Lupton (2006) argues for the importance of engaging with, and taking into account, lay understandings of risk rather than focusing on health status and health behaviour. Likewise we need further appreciation of these issues for health communication. Undoubtedly, understandings of risk are culturally defined and context dependent.

Additional impetus for understanding how health communication messages are interpreted and negotiated is rooted in what Bourne and Robson (2009: 285) refer to as the 'relative ineffectiveness' of health promotion strategies. There have also been calls by writers such as Chamberlain (2004) and Bunton (2006) to engage with more critical approaches within health psychology. The dominance of scientific, biomedical perspectives within health promotion and public health are less likely to take into account experience and meaning thus, as Bourne and Robson (2009) argue, health promotion strategies are likely to be rejected by the intended recipients who do not see their understandings and experiences reflected within them.

Given the challenges and critiques that have been outlined we turn to the position offered by critical health psychology. Critical health psychology challenges the natural science approach to health psychology which has traditionally resulted in the development of theoretical information processing and SCMs which attempt to predict or explain health behaviour (Willig, 2000). Critical perspectives challenge mainstream approaches within psychology in a number of ways. Experimental and quantitative methods of investigation are critiqued, as is the focus on the individual. Central to this is the challenge to the philosophical assumptions of mainstream psychology and a search for alternative positions. Critical health psychology gives attention to the social, political and cultural dimensions of health. The link between health promotion's philosophical foundations and radical roots should be apparent here. Given the limitations of the theories we have discussed we now turn to a critical consideration of the importance of context.

The importance of context

Much of the research on health behaviour has been dominated by positivist models which decontextualize experience and, as Pilkington (2007) argues, do not substantially consider socio-cultural context or wider influences on risk in health. It is important to try to understand the influence of socio-cultural context on health-related choices which, as Alexander et al. (2010) argue, is crucial to understanding risky health practices. In South Africa, for example, it is evident that patterns of substance use are inextricably bound up in the country's socio-political history. As Hendricks et al. (2015: 100) point out, 'decades of institutionalized racism, systematic oppression, social inequality, and the resulting context of low-income communities have been identified as the driving force behind high rates of substance use'. Yet approaches in mainstream health psychology have tended to focus on why people do not change their behaviour in response to risk communication (Lindsay, 2010).

A further criticism is levelled at the reductionist, deterministic focus of behaviour change theories. Similarly to the psychometric paradigm and cognitive theories, personality theories can be criticized for being reductionist, individualist and for ignoring (or downplaying) social contexts. However, it should be recognized that biopsychosocial approaches in health psychology do go some way to acknowledging the importance of social context (Sarafino and Smith, 2011). Certainly from a health promotion perspective the wider context is simply more important. Research into health behaviour to date has tended to focus on the value of different psychological theories for predicting health-related behaviour and testing assumptions that behaviour is mediated by cognitive processes (Connor and Norman, 2015). This focus on the individual inevitably leads to a victim-blaming approach (Green et al., 2015). At the very least we should consider the role that socio-economic circumstances play in health behaviour choices (Cockerham, 2005).

The importance of meaning: an example of risk-taking

We will use risk-taking to illustrate the importance of *meaning* in health communication. Mitchell et al. (2001) argue that it is important to take into account interpretations of risk and risk-taking practices as these give meaning to risk-taking in young people's lives. There are many studies which examine young people's risk perceptions (Austen, 2009); however, much of the research on risk does not consider its meaning (Boyne, 2003) nor, with regard to risky behaviours, does it seek to understand everyday 'ways of seeing' (Ioannou, 2005: 264). Instead research examines theoretical constructs in terms of their utility in predicting risky intentions or behaviours (Stainton-Rogers, 2012). As such, a significant amount of research within health psychology has examined the ways in which people perceive, respond to and manage risk. Risk perception is generally assumed to be a subjective judgement of the potential for harm or danger (Connor and Norman, 2015). However, writers such as Mielewczyk and Willig (2007) and Robertson and Williams (2010) advocate moving away from a focus on individual behavioural practices and the reliance on social cognition models to investigate 'health behaviours'. Instead, they argue that it is more important to further understanding of the meaning which certain practices have and the purposes or functions which they serve; in short, to increase understanding about why people behave in certain ways and engage in risk-taking (Cook and Bellis, 2001). As Denscombe (1993) argues, examining the meaning of risk-taking in health may offer crucial insight into apparent resistance to changing risky health behaviour.

Pidgeon et al. (2001) assert that mainstream psychological approaches to the study of risk, largely in the quantitative tradition, have resulted in valuable insights. However, the dominance of a positivist paradigm in risk research has led to the adoption of a 'deficit model'. The primary assumption within this is that people take risks because they do not understand the nature of risk, cannot make sense of it or are simply irrational (Tulloch and Lupton, 2003). Challenges to the deficit model can be seen in the turn towards an appreciation of *assets-based* and *salutogenic* approaches to health communication. Crossley (2002) offers a more agentic proposition, the notion of the rational actor who knowingly and deliberately takes risks. Parker and Stanworth (2005) take up this idea and argue that more attention should be paid to the notion of agency within risk research but this appears to be a relatively neglected area. Such ideas require further exploration and have implications for a range of issues such as policy-making and health communication.

The focus on rational decision-making processes results from an assumption that people are rational creatures who think through and consider alternatives in a logical fashion and who engage in a cost-benefit analysis before deciding on the best course of action (Stainton-Rogers, 2011). As illustrated earlier in this chapter, there are a range of models which are predicated on this assumption. Such models propose that individual perceptions of risk are paramount in determining the individual's intention to carry out a particular behaviour (Dillard et al., 2011). However, while the importance of risk perception in health-related behaviours is assumed to be apparent (Ancker et al., 2011) the predictive utility tends to be related to behavioural *intentions* rather than behavioural *outcomes*. Rhodes and de Bruijn (2013) carried out a systematic review and meta-analysis examining the intention-behaviour gap in relation to physical activity. They concluded that the focus on this is a weakness suggesting that additional constructs should be examined such as self-regulation and automaticity or that measurement of motivation should be improved.

Polič (2009) argues that individuals are not always candid about their conscious motivations and will not be aware of their unconscious ones. The role of emotion, though increasingly viewed as important, is also relatively neglected (Lawlor et al., 2003). However, interestingly, Weinstein et al. (2005) found that feelings about risk predicted behavioural outcomes more frequently than cognitions. Emotion and affect cover a range of human feelings which can and do have an effect on health behaviour. Note the example of comfort eating, which often originates from feelings of anxiety or boredom rather than from actually feeling hungry. A meta-analysis examined worry as an affective response to risk in health (Portnoy et al., 2014). This study found that worry was related to perceived susceptibility but was also distinguishable from it.

Implication for Practice 3

It is important to be aware of the limitations of different types of theory and to pay attention to the implications that these have for planning and evaluating health communication interventions. Different variables within different theories have different utility in relation to different issues. Critical understanding of available research is crucial. Applying what we know from the evidence base is also very important.

Behavioural ecological models

One of the key difficulties with the theories we have considered so far is that they are very much focused at the individual level. This can lead to victim-blaming, an approach we often see in practice but which, within health promotion, we would always strive to avoid.

Ecological models of behaviour set individual behaviour in context and give room for other factors to be considered and given more weight. Crucially ecological approaches acknowledge the inter-relationships between health, behaviour and their determinants high-lighting the complexity of health behaviours (Crosby et al., 2013b). One of the most influential ecological models has been the one pro-posed by Bronfenbrenner (1974). In this model, the environment outside the individual is seen as a critical factor in the determination of behaviour. The ecological model postulates that behaviour results from the interaction of five different levels as described by Kar et al. (2001b: 112).

1 *Intrapersonal factors* – individual characteristics, such as knowledge, attitudes, self-concept, skills, and developmental history
2 *Interpersonal factors* – relationships with primary social groups, including the family, peer networks, and the workplace (links to the discussion in the earlier section on 'the influence of others')
3 *Institutional factors* – social institutions with organizational char-acteristics, such as management styles, work schedules, and eco-nomic and social resources
4 *Community factors* – primary social groups to which an individual belongs, such as families, friendship networks, and neighbour-hoods, and relationships among social groups and organizations within a defined boundary
5 *Public policy* – local, state, and national laws and regulations that affect individual health

In order for behaviour change to occur, therefore, changes are needed in these levels. Such approaches give more weight to environmental and policy influences on behaviour change. After all, it is all very well to encourage people to cycle more but if roads are not safe to cycle on then this is a significant challenge to the individual cyclist. Using an ecological model to examine an issue enables the full complexity of the situation to be considered and moves the focus away from the behaviour of the individual. With regard to water, sanitation and hygiene in low-income countries Dreibelbis et al.'s (2013) systematic review shows that many different 'behavioural determinants' such as hand-washing and latrine use have been identified but that the role of the physical/natural environment had been relatively neglected. This has resulted in a 'profusion' of different theoretical frameworks or models specific to this significant public health issue (Dreibelbis et al., 2013: 1018). Crucially, however, from a health promotion perspective, they found that several factors were under-accounted for in many of the models such as the type of water and sanitation technology and the cost and complexity of using it. Contextual factors such as socio-economic status, the physical environment and resource availability were also under-represented. In order to address the inherent limitations of existing frameworks, drawing on research in Bangladesh, Dreibelbis et al. (2013) propose a new theory – the Integrated Behavioural Model for Water, Sanitation, and Hygiene (IBM-WASH) – 'to provide both a conceptual and practical tool for improving understanding and evaluation of the multi-level, multi-dimensional factors that influence water, sanitation, and hygiene practices in infrastructure-constrained settings' (p. 1016).

Changes in our environment can and do cause changes to our individual behaviour. Ecological models view behaviour as resulting from the interaction between internal factors and environmental (external) factors (Hayden, 2014). They therefore sit nicely within an agenda focused on the social determinants of health. Tackling the social determinants of health is another concern which is central to health promotion philosophy and practice. Through the creation of supportive environments behaviour change may be effected. The importance of multi-level and structural level approaches is therefore apparent. For example, tackling obesity may only be possible by using an ecological approach which would include addressing the factors in all five levels (Crosby et al., 2013a; 2013b).

Theory of triadic influence

The theory of triadic influence adapts and develops ideas from Bronfenbrenner's ecological model and from social learning theory (Crosby et al., 2013b) in order to explain behaviour and behaviour change (Flay, 1999). It proposes three streams of influence:

1 *Intrapersonal (personal) stream* – this includes constructs such as self-control, self-efficacy and competence
2 *Interpersonal (social) stream* – this includes influences on behavioural norms that come from family, work and friends
3 *Socio-cultural environment (environmental) stream* – this includes influences such as the media, social organization and culture

Alongside the three streams the theory proposes three different levels of causation – ultimate, distal and proximal (Bavarian et al.,

2014). The ultimate level refers to causes that people have little control over; the distal level refers to causes that people have some control over and the proximal level refers to causes that are seen to be under people's control (Snyder and Flay, 2012). When the three streams of influence are combined with the three different levels of causation a matrix is produced whereby health communication and health promotion efforts may be targeted in any of nine different areas. A recent longitudinal study carried out in South Korea by Chun (2015) used the theory of triadic influence to examine smoking in female adolescents. The study concluded that social factors at all three levels of causation influenced smoking patterns. Specifically the analysis showed that several factors influenced smoking practices. These were 'parental supervision, attachment to friends, peer smoking prevalence, stigma, attitude towards smoking, self-control and stress' (Chun, 2015: 85). A cursory glance at the literature shows that the theory of triadic influence has been sparingly applied in research into behaviour and behaviour as compared with the 'classic' theories presented earlier in this chapter. Despite the potential for using this model in a different way to try to understand behaviour, researchers who have used it also had recourse to the individualistic, reductionist and positivist approaches that have been critiqued in this chapter. There is perhaps an opportunity to use this theory in a more creative way and to use more qualitative means of investigation.

The focus on behavioural intention is also still apparent in this theory. We need to move away from focusing on individual characteristics and behavioural intention as assumed precursors to behaviour given their relatively limited predictive usefulness and the fact that such approaches reflect a very limited approach to effecting change. As argued, we need to develop alternative approaches to understanding. Golden and Earp (2012: 364) drive this point home. In a review of twenty years of papers on health promotion interventions published in the journal *Health Education and Behavior* they found that 'overall, articles were more likely to describe interventions focused on individual and interpersonal characteristics, rather than institutional, community, or policy factors'. They concluded that there is a need to focus on improvements to health through social and political environments instead. This is illustrated very well by a paper arguing for a behavioural ecological approach to teenage pregnancy in the UK which concludes 'the attempt to reduce teenage pregnancy rates through simple proximate correlates, health concerns or moral issues is unlikely to be successful if young women continue to live in poverty or perceive their environment as being hazardous, have experiences in their family or neighbourhood that truncate their future expectations, and, in consequence, make the reproductive decision to start having their children at a young age' (Dickens et al., 2012: 356). A qualitative study carried out in Israel, which used the behavioural ecological model to explore why the ban on smoking in public places implemented in 2007 had only been partially successful, found that social norms supporting smoking were influential. The authors concluded that changing social norms through targeted health communication efforts was necessary (Baron-Epel et al., 2012).

Despite the complexity of such approaches (Dresler-Hawke and Whitehead, 2009), the behavioural ecological model (and similar theoretical frameworks) is much more akin to health promotion's central concern with social determinants of health than the classic models of behaviour change we discussed earlier in this chapter. Behaviour and behaviour change is complex so any theory which attempts to explain or understand these will be necessarily complex. In addition, there is also a relative paucity of research using behavioural ecological approaches, as pointed out by Gubbels et al. (2014) who lament the lack of empirical research 'operationalizing a true ecological view in diet and physical activity'. In their research conducted in this area with children in the Netherlands they conclude that this might be for a number of reasons including complexity and publication bias. They call for more studies applying an ecological approach citing Ding and Gebel (2012) whose umbrella review of 36 reviews on the influence of the physical environment on physical activity 'revealed that the most cited suggestion for future research was to examine moderators of environmental influences' (Gubbels et al., 2014: 65).

> ## Implication for Practice 4
>
> Interventions based on ecological approaches to behaviour change reflect a more complex, yet nuanced approach to human behaviour and are more likely to be effective. Efforts to promote behaviour change should not be limited to those focused at an individual level, should be multipronged and should be aimed at addressing factors that affect behaviour at different levels.

In conclusion, it has long been argued that behaviour change interventions should be underpinned by theory, yet it is acknowledged that there are many instances where this is not the case and that there are inconsistencies in the literature (Prestwich et al., 2013). Indeed,

Prestwich et al.'s (2013) systematic review of physical activity and dietary interventions which analysed 140 interventions based on two theories – Social Cognitive Theory and the TTM – concluded that using them more extensively is unlikely to increase intervention effectiveness. Arguably, if there is little or no impact on effectiveness, this would appear to undermine arguments for a strong theoretical foundation; nevertheless there are those that firmly advocate such an approach (Green et al., 2015). There is a more recent focus in health psychology on deconstructing and reconstructing the more 'traditional' models of behaviour change and producing taxonomies of behaviour change techniques led by Professor Susan Michie (Michie et al., 2010). This has resulted in the development of the behaviour change wheel (see Michie et al., 2011). The overall critique presented in this chapter should still be taken into consideration with regard to such developments; nevertheless, they are an indication of how theoretical knowledge and understanding about behaviour change is developing and has the potential to impact on practice in health communication.

Summary of key points

This chapter has provided a critical overview of behaviour change theory deriving from the discipline of psychology. Specifically it has:

- given a brief overview of several 'classic' theories of behaviour change
- examined key concepts in psychological theory such as the influence of others, self-esteem and notions of control
- presented a generic critique of behaviour change theory originating in psychology
- considered the importance of context and meaning for health behaviour and the implications for health communication
- introduced some alternative approaches to understanding health behaviour

> **Reflection 1** – There are many more theories of behaviour change in the literature in addition to the ones discussed in this chapter. Try to find out some information about one or two different theories and how they have been used in the health communication research. Identify the key concepts within them and the usefulness of these. What does the research say about effectiveness?

Reflection 2 – As we have established within the chapter, theories of behaviour change are open to criticism. Building on what you did in the first reflection think about what are the potential limitations of the theories you have chosen. How might these limitations be taken into account in practice?

Reflection 3 – Following on from Reflection 3 how do you think our understanding of health behaviour might be improved? What would we need to take into account and how could we do this? What implications will this have for health communication efforts? At what level do you think efforts should be directed and why? i.e. Policy? Structural? Environmental?

Reflection 4 – How might behavioural ecological theories enhance our understanding of health behaviour? How might such understanding underpin more effective interventions for health communication? What is the potential use of behavioural ecological theories in the context in which you work?

Further reading

Connor, M. and Norman, P. (2015) *Predicting and Changing Health Behaviour.* 3rd edn. Maidenhead: Open University Press.

This book provides a carefully detailed chapter by chapter consideration of the 'classic' behaviour change theories referenced briefly in this chapter. Each theory is presented in turn and evaluated in relation to relevant literature and research.

DiClemente, R. J., Salazar, L. F. and Crosby, R. A. (2013) *Health Behaviour Theory for Public Health: Principles, Foundations, and Applications.* Burlington, MA: Jones and Barlett Learning.

This text provides a broad overview of a range of theories relevant to health communication and public health.

Stainton-Rogers, W. (2011) *Social Psychology.* 2nd edn. Maidenhead: McGraw-Hill Open University Press.

This accessible textbook on social psychology complements the contents of this chapter nicely. It takes a critical perspective on a range of issues raised in this chapter.

Part II

Key Topics

5

Methods and Media

Key aims

- To present and discuss mass media communication in health and related theoretical perspectives such as Diffusion of Innovation
- To consider the use of mass media for advocacy
- To examine the evidence base for the effectiveness of various methods of communication such as emotional appeal and peer education
- To analyse the development of electronic and social media for communication such as the internet, the use of mobile phones and text messaging

Introduction

Health messages can be communicated to the public individually, in small groups or to a mass audience. In Part I of this book, we examined a range of communication, education and psychological theories that underpin health communication. We also examined the skills of the communicator in interpersonal communication, the need to be self-aware and reflective in order to communicate effectively. This chapter will focus further on the practical aspects of health communication, particularly focusing on mass communication and other approaches to the diffusion, discussion and dissemination of health messages. We will explore various methods and media in communicating health messages, focusing on the channel, the media and message of the communication loop, the vehicle and the way health messages are communicated to the public, bringing together interpersonal communication skills and knowledge of mass communication and how they can complement each other.

Mass communication

Mass communication is about communicating messages to a mass audience via a medium such as television, newspaper, internet ... whereas mass media refers to the media that are designed to reach a large audience and where mass communication takes place. In practice, mass communication, mass media, mass media communication are terms that are often used interchangeably. Mass communication mainly developed as a social phenomenon in the twentieth century. It symbolized industrialization and the struggle of democracy and conflicts of the twentieth century (McQuail, 2010). Early verbal and printed media used in disseminating information to large audiences grew rapidly before and during the Second World War. After the war, mass communication continued to grow in scale and increasing diversity as electronic media continued to expand. However, the effectiveness of mass communication has been continuously debated as the large-scale, one-way, top-down information transfer, via traditional methods and media such as megaphone approaches, posters and billboards, leaflets, newspaper, radio, television, continued to grow into a new era of social media. The transformation of globalized networks and the speed of information transfer would have been unimaginable twenty years ago. The development of new technologies has blurred the lines between private and public communication. It has also blurred the lines between interpersonal and mass communication. Ours is a networked world where decision-making is based on complex connections of information. The discussion about mass communication is about time, context and power where the speed of information, when and where it's produced are important. It's also about its power over the audience even where attention to mass media seems voluntary and appears to be a personal choice (McQuail, 2010).

Corcoran (2013) identified four different categories of mass media in mass communication. The most widely used media are:

1 audio-visual broadcast media such as television, radio, advertisements, news items, debates, documentaries;
2 audio-visual non-broadcast media such as videos, CDs, DVDs;
3 print media such as newspapers, magazines, leaflets and posters, journals, books, mail shots, billboards;

4 electronic media such as the internet – websites, search engines, YouTube and mobile phones.

However, classifying approaches within these four categories can seem simplistic. Health Communication practice is much more fluid. Some approaches cut across a number of categories. Others will use a combination of mass communication and interpersonal communication to maximize their effect, to reinforce information provision, clarifying messages and stimulating discussion. This chapter's starting point will be what one might describe as classic broadcasting or mass communication, mainly seen in audio-visual broadcasting and print media, mainly top-down, mainly one-way, which could be seen as paternalistic, towards more interpersonal approaches and interactive processes where power is discussed and shared, and where newer technologies shift the conversation.

The effectiveness of mass communication

The use of mass media in mass communication can have a wide and rapid reach and be a powerful agent of communication. Mass communication is also very popular in health promotion, being relatively low cost per head (Wakefield et al., 2010). However, its cost-effectiveness is more contested (Wellings and Macdowall, 2000), in terms of firstly the actual change that mass communication can bring about, secondly the complexity of change, negative and positive, in terms of healthy behaviour and thirdly the paternalistic agendas which can underpin mass communication campaigns. A review by Wakefield et al. (2010) concluded that mass media campaigns can promote behaviour changes if a combination of interventions is used. It also works better if it is one-off or episodic. The availability of adequate resources to support behaviour changes is also essential. It is unrealistic to expect changes when the facilities and help are not available to support changes. The use of mass media in communication also has limitations in conveying complex information, teaching skills, in shifting attitudes and beliefs, and in changing behaviour in the absence of enabling factors (Wellings and Macdowall, 2000). Mass communication works better when there are limited oppositional and counter-messages. It also works better with the support of interpersonal communication. Lazarsfeld and Merton (1955) noted there are three conditions for mass media effectiveness:

Monopolization where messages are consistent with the audience's existing motivations and/or plug into existing prejudices, desires and wishes, telling people what they want to hear;

Canalization where they are supplemented and supported by interpersonal influences;

Supplementation where supporting programmes centre on interpersonal interaction.

Successful outcomes in mass communication campaigns can be difficult to demonstrate with many complex influences and conflicting messages around. Potentially, but not inevitably, mass communication campaigns can make a difference. In the health field, 75 per cent of people claim they rely on media coverage when making health decisions (Barker et al., 2006). Information from the media can have a powerful influence on public perceptions of health issues. Mass media is often used to educate the public and to influence behaviour changes, to encourage people in making healthy choices. For example, Vallone et al. (2011) recommended the US Government in providing funding for mass media campaigns involving smoking cessation. Webb et al. (2011) also suggested that conventional mass media campaigns can engage an extra 6 per cent of people in stair-climbing activities in mall settings. Indeed, we started this in our University where posters have been placed in front of lifts to encourage staff and students to use the stairs to the first three floors. In all of these, the audience is passive (Wakefield et al., 2010). Health promotion, on the other hand, is about prompting active thought, even in a passive audience as discussed in Chapter 2. Audience motivation is needed for change to take place. The communicator needs to know how to motivate people, stimulate bottom-up information processing in the audience. An audience involved with the topic needs to seek, attend to and process health messages actively (Maibach and Parrott, 1995).

The assumptions underpinning mass media communication can also be problematic. At times it can produce unhelpful 'noise' or even undermine empowering change. Current mass media approaches can assume the individual to be the sole focus to be addressed, often seen in many television campaigns on lifestyle such as smoking, drinking and healthy eating. Commercial interests can also use the same mass media to promote unhealthy influences, behaviour or products. Consumerist health can seem to sell health products or top-down behaviour change rather than empowering the public to make healthy, perhaps non-consumerist choices (Green et al., 2015).

There is often a focus on the responsibility of the individual and a failure to address underlying political and social causes. The social and environmental causes of ill-health can also be seen through a medical lens. This 'victim-blaming' message can become even more explicit in the media. For example, issues are often presented as 'infotainment' ('Benefits Street', 'Embarrassing Bodies') where the viewer is invited (at best) to gaze at these strange people or (at worst) blame them for their problems and our taxes. Mass media approaches can also focus on emotional appeals and shock tactics, regularly showing images on television, photos on posters and leaflets, undermining change or even building up resistance to change. One of the key discussion points later in this chapter will be about the use of appeals, where the strategy is to seek out an emotional response and can be very emotionally charged.

Implication for Practice 1

Mass media communication is potentially very powerful in communicating health messages. However, there is a need to think about limitations when you choose mass communication methods in the development of your health promotion campaign.

From paternalism to interpersonal communication

As we have seen, mass communication tends to be a one-way and top-down communication method, missing any meaningful feedback, as seen in Lasswell's formula in Chapter 2. It is often a paternalistic approach with society being the passive subject of an intervention. Modern mass communication does attempt to include feedback in his communication strategy. Comments can be sent via phone-ins or written in via e-mail and Twitter, or debated in a forum. However, it is often unclear how (or, indeed, if) these comments make a difference to the strategy. Direct feedback is very limited.

One of the earlier mass media models is the *'Direct Effect'* model where messages are 'injected' into the individual like a hypodermic needle or magic bullet effect as critically discussed by Klapper (1966) and Berger (1995). It can have a strategic approach to change but remains paternalistic. The theory is consistent with earlier mass communication campaigns when mass media had a direct and powerful effect on the passive audience. Mendelsohn (1968) discredited this magic bullet theory and saw mass media as like an *aerosol spray*.

Some hits the target, but most drifts and very little penetrates. He questioned the power of mass media in the effectiveness of behaviour change. Katz and Lazarsfeld (1955), in their development of the two-step model, showed that people are not passive recipients of information. The two-step model stresses the importance of interpersonal communication. Opinion leaders act as change agents, strengthening the message, mass media information is channelled via opinion leaders to the wider population. The influence of change agents promotes the reception of messages. This laid the foundation for the study of Diffusion of Innovation.

Diffusion of Innovation originated from Rogers and is also known as Communication of Innovation (Rogers and Shoemaker, 1971). This is a social change theory describing how information diffuses to the public, a process by which information passes systemically through certain channels over time (Rogers, 2003). There are five stages in the adoption process.

1 Knowledge is communicated;
2 the public develops awareness and understanding;
3 persuasion, when a favourable attitude is formed and the decision is made;
4 the innovation is put into practice; and
5 uptake is confirmed.

Graphically, the adoption process follows an S-shaped pattern – a slow initial rate from the innovators to the early adopters, then there is a surge of the early majority, and the late majority, and finally the process then slows down when saturation occurs with some laggards left behind. There are four key essential elements associated with the uptake of innovation – the characteristic of innovation, the communication channel, the time and rate of the adoption and the social system itself. It stresses the important role of the change agent since adopters can become change agents themselves and continue to influence friends through an interpersonal approach. The message also becomes stronger when adopters become change agents (Rogers, 2003).

Peer education and community art

Peer education and community art are two communication methods which can be used as examples to show how interpersonal communication enhances mass media strategy. *Peer Education* is a very popular method, particularly in sexual health among young people. It is a useful way to influence and promote behaviour change (UNAIDS, 1999). As seen in the two-step model above, peer educators can act as change agents when working with their clients and help to reinforce and clarify health messages in the media, thus promoting a positive attitude towards accepting the innovation and enhancing the effectiveness of mass communication messages.

Apart from school settings, peer-based approaches to promoting health are also widely used, for example, in prison within the criminal justice system (Green et al., 2015). Although the evidence is patchy, Wright et al. (2011) in their systematic review demonstrated positive outcomes in sexual health and substance abuse in prison resulting from peer education. It is also widely used in African countries such as Zambia (Burke et al., 2012). Peer educators from the same societal group educate each other and become change agents and reinforce the health messages in the public domain. We can easily be influenced by people similar to ourselves (Windahl et al., 2009). An evaluation of five Youth Peer Education programmes in Zambia (Svenson et al., 2008) shows that the highest quality programme was also the most expensive overall and per peer educator trained. They also spent the longest hours working on programme activities and made the largest number of contacts. The higher quality programme does promote HIV knowledge, increased intentions to use condoms, lower stigma and discrimination towards people living with HIV/ AIDS, increased likelihood of using a condom and the use of sexual health related services by highly vulnerable youth. Appropriate referrals were also made by peer educators.

Recruitment of peer educators is an important aspect. Peer educators tend to be self-selected volunteers or approached by the health promotion project co-coordinator or the teacher if it is a school setting. Mason-Jones et al. (2011) looked at the selection and recruitment of peer educators in a school environment in a study in South Africa. This indicated that they are higher achievers and less socially disadvantaged as compared with their peer group. The *'peerness'* and *'connectedness'* (Mason-Jones et al., 2011: 69) is important in the selection of peer educators and needs further investigation. The importance of peer educators is that they live in the same cultural and socio-economic and political context as their peers. They understand the challenges within that specific context and their equal status helps avoid professional-client power relationships. Peer educators selected should be accepted and respected by the group. Their information needs to be credible to act as role models to facilitate the shifting of social norms within their peer group. For this reason, peer education can be particularly useful and acceptable for the so-called 'hard-to-reach' groups in the community.

Peer education is a social process. One of the questions about it is its sustainability. A process evaluation of a project on young people and sexual health in a school in Scotland by Backett-Milburn and Wilson (2000) showed the challenges that peer education methods encounter. In a school environment, the selection of peer educators resembled passing an academic hurdle. The role of coordinator is varied and demanding, from organizing the project initially, recruitment of peer educators, training and support, relationship negotiation between peer educators and the teacher as well as responsibility for its future development. There are also difficulties both at operational level in a school setting and at the cultural level about how schools are run as compared with how health promotion works. Young peer educators are aware of the approaches that they can use to maximize the effectiveness of their health messages to suit the needs of their audience. They gained skills in communicating health, negotiating the power relationships with their own peers and the knowledge of the topic itself. There is also a question of adult control and trust. Peer educators need to be trusted to do the job. Young people grow up quickly, leave school and move on after a few years. So recruitment and training are continuous. On-going support and training is needed for it to be successful and effective.

Methods that mean most to people themselves and that they are most comfortable with will have a greater success; for example, bottom-up approaches in community development such as *Community Art* can have dramatic and sustainable effects. Examples of such methods are drama, songs, storytelling, arts projects ... These interpersonal communication methods can increase social cohesion, community support networks and thereby community capital (Dixey et al., 2013). They can be complementary to mass communication e.g. using non-broadcasting mass communication materials such as videos, CDs, posters and leaflets as tools in health promotion activities. The community workers can also act as change agents helping to clarify and strengthen health messages in the media. For example, many of our African students and health promotion colleagues write and use drama scripts to stimulate discussions on public health issues in the media and in the community.

Carson et al. (2007) discussing the promotion of health through a community art centre suggested that such a centre can be grounded within an ecological health promotion model and add value in the delivery of traditional health promotion activities. Community art can help to build community capacity and social capital, enhancing individual well-being and help develop and regenerate communities. Taylor et al. (2012) studied the use of role play to reduce teenage pregnancy in a school-based programme. They found that role play is effective in information giving, modelling behaviour and developing interpersonal skills. It has the potential for building self-efficacy among learners with respect to sexual behaviour. Role play can be used to challenge perspectives in environments where patriarchy is dominant. However, training of educators is needed to increase the sustainability of these programmes.

The use of mass media in communicating health messages

Television and radio transmission are two of the most common media for mass communication, particularly accessible for people with low reading skills. Television reaches large audiences. Radio transmission is very useful if people are mobile or in rural areas where there is a poor television signal or are, for example, travelling in the car. Communicating health information via programmes such as soap operas on television and radio can be very effective. They mirror audiences' construction of reality and focus on common concerns (Green et al., 2015). Similarly, celebrities can also be used to raise important public health issues. Brown and De Matviuk (2010) discussed sports celebrity Diego Maradona and his effect on drug abuse in Argentina particularly among young people. Celebrities may provide a means of social influence. For example, Jade Goody's story in the UK had a dramatic effect on the uptake of cervical cancer screening. Jamie Oliver on healthy eating and healthy school meals is another example, raising awareness of healthy eating among school children as well as raising awareness among policy makers.

Activities labelled as enter-educate, edutainment, entertainment-education, infotainment have emerged (Windahl et al., 2009) and can be useful in sensitive issues such as sexual health. Audiences can be receptive both emotionally and intellectually. Television and radio programmes, comics, books are all potential media for this. Effectiveness can also increase if supplemented by messages from an integrated campaign (Windahl et al., 2009). However, there is a need for the entertainment industry to work with health promoters to maximize the effects. According to the *Elaboration Likelihood Model*, media messages are processed through a central route or superficial route in an individual. An audience will critically think about the message if it is processed via a central route. Messages will be accepted or discarded without much elaboration if they are processed through a superficial route (McQuail, 2010). Therefore the design of messages is important in order to enable the audience to process the message critically and decide if it is accepted, resulting in a change of behaviour and attitude. Similarly, this can also explain the usefulness of entertainment such as dramas and soap operas for health promotion purposes. Audiences choose what they like to watch and such means may be a source of advice and support.

Emotional appeal in mass communication

Emotional appeals, such as shock tactics, are commonly used as persuasive devices in public health. Fear appeals use images to show health consequences e.g. in sexual health. Their effectiveness is, however, debatable. Turner (2012) discussed guilt appeal such as smoking that harms a baby; anger appeal such as anger to pressurize the government on policies often seen in the media about, for example, refugees and migrants; humorous appeals to connect positive feelings to issues being addressed. She suggested the failure of emotional appeal is usually due to a lack of engagement with the audience and the message not striking a chord; the message can be overly intense, causing defensiveness; or feelings of inappropriateness for the audience. According to Rogers' *Protection Motivation Theory* (Rogers, 1975), people make cognitive assessments of the threat and decide what actions to take to address the problem. The concept was further developed in the area of persuasive communication (Rogers, 1983). Based on the threat appraisal and coping appraisal, an evaluation can be made in regard to actions and strategies. Hence it is important to provide information on action about how to eliminate a certain threat to minimize the maladaptive response.

There are also ethical dilemmas concerning the acceptability of persuasive communication as well as the actual threat made to the public. From a deontological perspective, all public health measures must be grounded in a priori moral certainties, the absolute moral foundation. Based on the principle of beneficence, deontologists would reject approaches that instil anxiety, distress and guilt as an attack on public mental well-being regardless of the ultimate societal gains. On the other hand, a teleological perspective focuses on outcomes and accepts the action as being ultimately beneficial for public health; the good ends justify the means (Bradley, 2011). From the utilitarian's point of view, it is acceptable to sacrifice the rights of a few for the greatest good for the greatest number of people. All of this raises complex questions about the relationship between the state and the individuals and organizations affected by policies (Nuffield Council on Bioethics, 2007). The stewardship model, based on John Stuart Mill's Harm Principles, sets out guiding principles for making decisions about public health policies. The 'intervention ladder' provides a way of thinking about the acceptability of different public health measures. The use of power and persuasion to guide public health action, based on the greater good, can be portrayed as paternalistic.

Implication for Practice 2

Think about your practice, do you use emotional appeals and attempts to persuade your clients when designing communication campaigns? Do they have the resources and adequate information to make the change?

We live in an information-rich and media-driven society. Ratzan (2011b) discussed health-related information and referred to 'TMI' – Too Much Information. Functionalist sociology sees the media as serving societal needs, for example for cultural continuity, social cohesion and social control. The media reacts to the needs of the population e.g. the need for information, entertainment and relaxation (McQuail, 2010). Contemporary audiences are transformed into active participants. According to *Uses and Gratification Theory*, individuals interact and select media messages that suit their own needs and align with their own values and beliefs (Blumler and Katz, 1974; McQuail, 2010). People's motives derive from their needs, e.g. for orientation, security, interaction and tension-release. McQuail et al.'s (1972) typology of media-person interactions suggested the audience has a need for information seeking; for diversion, an escape from routine and problems; a need for personal relationships, learning to relate to others and a need for personal identity in self-reference and reinforcement of personal values.

Media advocacy and narrowcasting

As noted above, mass media can focus on coaxing the individual to change. However, one useful function of mass media is in the development of healthy public policy through public debate. Media advocacy helps to refocus the responsibility for health from the individual onto social, political and environmental changes. It aligns with empowerment approaches and values of health promotion (Green et al., 2015). Healthy public policy is an action area in the Ottawa Charter (WHO, 1986) and advocacy is a key strategy in building such healthy public policy. Media advocacy is a strategic use of mass media to shape agendas and debates in public health issues, mobilize communities to influence policy makers in decision-making, prioritize health and promote community development. It is about seeking policy solutions to tackle health issues (Dorfman and Krasnow, 2014). It is a promising complementary strategy to conventional media campaigns (Wakefield et al., 2010). As health promoters aiming to bring about social justice in health (Beauchamp, 1976; Cross et al., 2013), it is our responsibility to put health promotion on the social agenda in a democratic society.

Upstream approaches to health promotion are about tackling the physical, social and political environment surrounding the individual, influencing the social, economic and political factors affecting health. Media advocacy is a social justice tool for public health practitioners, attempting to address social determinants of health. On a superficial level, mass communication is about using mass media for public information and education, a paternalistic way of promoting health. It also assumes that each individual is equally empowered to accept or reject these messages, in line with a neoliberal paradigm. Implicitly, poor health is the individual's choice and fault. Media advocacy, on the other hand, helps to refocus the function of health communication. It's about raising awareness of health issues, with system change (rather than individual behaviour) as the starting point. It uses mass media in its most powerful form to foster a democratic process for people to participate in decision-making, for cxample using individual stories to put health issues on the agenda, opening up discussion (Dorfman and Krasnow, 2014), raising public concerns and forcing the government to take action. In narrowcasting, messages are sent to a specific group of people or individuals, for example targeted policy makers, industry directors (Green et al., 2015) aiming at influencing changes at policy and structural levels rather than individual behaviour change. Media advocacy is a good example of where communities use mass media in an empowering way to promote health.

Social media and digital technologies

Modern technology can enable health services to become more accessible and efficient (DH, 2012). Interpersonal and mediated communication channels can complement each other in health-related contexts using modern technologies (Hou and Shim, 2010). According to Fox and Jones (2009), 61 per cent of American adults seek health information from the internet. Although most campaign designers use traditional communication methods for health promotion, there has been a gradual increase in the use of interactive technologies over the last decade (Atkin and Rice, 2013). In this section, we view social media as an internet-based interactive platform where interactive Web 2.0 technologies are being used for users to generate content, share and exchange information, participate in social networking, for example Facebook, Twitter, blogs, WhatsApp, Instagram . . . It also has to be said that since social media is a fast moving industry, the discussion here may become out of date quickly.

Internet information tends to be user-led rather than provider-led. People seeking internet-based health information are usually looking for disease specific information. An unsatisfactory (face-to-face) consultation motivates people to seek information (e.g.) on the internet. Koch-Weser et al. (2010) looked at a range of studies and found that internet health information seekers tend to be women, White, less than sixty years of age, with higher incomes and educational attainment. Those who go to the web first before seeking professional help tend to be younger, better educated and with a higher income. There were, however, no differences in gender and race. Hou and Shim (2010) found that there is a high level of trust in internet health information. Their findings suggested that the internet has become an important source of health information, even for middle-aged people.

The use of social media is particularly important for young people (Centre for Health Promotion and Women's and Children's Health Network, 2012; Gold et al., 2012; Loss et al., 2013). According to the Centre for Health Promotion Women's and Children's Health Network in South Australia (2012), nine out of ten sixteen- to twenty-nine-year-olds use the internet daily and spend more time online than any other groups, while young children aged eight to eleven years are likely to play games on the computer, those aged twelve to seventeen are more interested in social networking. In a systematic review by Martin et al. (2011) on the use of a variety of networked communication technologies on mental health conditions in young people, networked communication seemed to reduce symptoms and complications and improve patient and healthcare professional encounters. However, the quality of transmission with these technologies was a concern. There were also concerns about confidentiality and privacy about whether these technologies can complement or enhance face-to-face consultation for specific patients.

There has been a dramatic increase in the amount of information available on the internet, with scientifically valid data and evidence-based recommendations. There is also more poor quality data, personal opinions, anecdotes and misinformation (Ratzan, 2011a). Online health information searches do not replace health professionals as an information source (Fox and Jones, 2009), but are an additional resource to complement consultation with physicians (Stevenson et al., 2007). Ahmad et al. (2006) found that physicians believed online information often led to patient misinformation, confusion, distress, or harmful self-diagnosis and self-treatment. As digital technologies grow, health practitioners need to direct clients towards the more useful online information sites related to their treatment, lifestyles and emotional needs, and to discuss with health professionals the health information they obtained (Hou and Shim, 2010). As the evidence base in the use of social media develops, there is a responsibility and need for collaboration among leaders of different sectors to build an ethical, theoretical, scientific and evidence-based foundation to advance accurate information and knowledge (Ratzan, 2011b).

Atkin and Salmon (2010) found that the use of interactive technologies in the USA is still sporadic. A range of digital media techniques were used in healthcare such as interactiveness, narrowcasting via audience segmentation, targeting internet users and tailoring messages to create publicity and raise the profile of the campaign embedding campaigns into entertainment programmes . . . They also found that the internet can be used to provide social support groups, improve quality of life and increase self-efficacy. The anonymity in web information is also welcome for sensitive topics. Well-designed campaigns with online mentors, e-mail and interpersonal support can also provide better support for young people (Rhodes et al., 2006). Digital media with only a simple banner is less successful whereas paid adverts in social media sites with prominent placement and precisely targeted messages are more successful (Atkin and Rice, 2013). Campaigns which are underpinned by theories are also more successful (Webb et al., 2010). Other technologies such as blogs, Twitter and podcast can also be used to update followers, although Scanfeld et al. (2010) found that tweets can be a cause of misunderstanding and abuse of health information.

Whiting and Williams (2013) identified ten uses and gratifications for using social media. Their study showed 88 per cent for social interaction, 80 per cent for information seeking, 76 per cent for pastimes, 64 per cent for entertainment, 60 per cent for relaxation, 56 per cent for communicatory utility, 56 per cent for expressing opinions, 52 per cent for convenience utility, 40 per cent for information sharing and 20 per cent for surveillance and watching others. Although it provides an insight into the appeal of health information, it also shows the audience is not a passive one, in a modern representation of the aerosol spray theory and the limitations of the hypodermic needles effect of mass communication (Green et al., 2015). It also demonstrates the limitations of many mass media methods such as newspapers, television and radio as health promotion media. People only choose certain newspapers, certain television channels, complicating any strategies of the health promoters.

Bennett and Glasgow (2009: 274) described the increased use of Web 2.0 technologies as an 'indispensable communication tool'. It can be seen as two-way communication with interaction and collaboration between the people involved. Ratzan (2011c) agreed about the opportunity to leverage these new communication technologies and tools for public health. People also actively used websites to manage their lifestyles. Thus, the internet can be viewed as a promising way for the public to gradually develop ownership of their own health (Hou and Shim, 2010). The UK has a very strong platform for present and future digital potential. A holistic approach is required of government, businesses and the community. Resources are needed to improve infrastructure and the engagement of individuals and organizations. Innovation and entrepreneurship of private and non-profit-making companies is also needed (Koss et al., 2012). According to Booz and Company, a global management consulting firm (Koss et al., 2012), universal digitization can have substantial economic and social benefits, encourage social changes for individuals, small and medium size enterprises, charities and government.

In the UK, the NHS digital strategy (Lafferty, 2013) aims to give its staff the knowledge, skills, permission and confidence to embrace digital technology in the delivery of better care and better health. In a speech to Policy Exchange (DH, 2013a), the then Health Secretary, Jeremy Hunt set out 'The Digital Challenge' in the NHS and announced that the NHS would go paperless by 2018, saying that this would save billions of pounds, improve services and help meet the healthcare needs of our ageing population. A study by Price Waterhouse Coopers found that measures such as the use of text messaging, electronic prescribing and electronic patient records could help to save money and improve care by allowing health professionals to spend more time with patients (DH, 2013a). The internet can also be used as an online platform for healthcare practitioners to facilitate conference discussions and networking. It is similar in the Public Health arena where the use of the internet in health communication is a common strategy. Hunt (2013) said that 'The NHS cannot be the last man standing as the rest of the economy embraces the technology revolution. Only with world-class information systems will the NHS deliver world-class care'. The need to enhance health literacy to ensure significant health outcomes in this digital age is apparent (Kickbusch et al., 2013) as can be seen in Chapter 7 on Health Literacy.

Digital literacy is increasingly important in education for a digitally competent workforce and can improve employability for healthcare practitioners (Sharpe et al., 2010). There is an organizational need for healthcare practitioners to be proficient in the use of digital technologies at work (Pawlyn, 2012), and for health promoters to communicate health messages. The paper from the NHS-HE Connectivity Best Practice Working Group of the NHS-HE Forum (Lafferty, 2013) provides recommendations to healthcare staff and University colleagues on the use of Web 2.0 technologies. The paper also identified risks in using social media, including possible breach of patient confidentiality and copyright, cyber-bullying and lapses in professionalism.

Siemens (2005) argues that there is a need to evaluate traditional learning theories in a digital era. Behaviourism, cognitivism and constructivism attempt to address how individuals learn. However, they address the actual learning process, but not the effectiveness of what is being learned. Siemens believes learning should focus on connections, a process of connecting information sources. The public needs to develop the ability to filter the continuous flow of incoming information to make decisions in this networked world. Connectivism is an alternative theory of learning in the digital age where connections of information sources are important – the connection of the nodes. It plays an important role where learners are increasingly gaining control of their learning. The internet has changed communication towards a more 'horizontal' dialogue-based form of communication. This change in the way people learn, think and communicate is reshaping the ways in which health information needs to be communicated (Ratzan, 2011b).

Mobile phones and text messaging

Text messaging using mobile phones is a relatively simple, but a very common form of social communication. Mobile phones and short text services are better suited for tailored and interactive messaging (Fjeldsoe et al., 2009). 67 per cent of the world's population own a mobile phone. 75 per cent of cell phone owners reported regularly sending and receiving text messages (Kohut et al., 2012). Lenhart (2010) found that 65 per cent of cell phone owners sleep with their phone in or next to their bed; this is an integral part of people's lives. Text messaging is also important for people who don't have television or internet access.

Hazelwood (2008) used a mobile phone text messaging service for her clients with eating disorders, irrespective of their age. Her clients could text her anytime and this seemed to be a positive thing, offering the client the reassurance of therapist availability. It allowed the therapist to construct a careful and planned reply. Her clients were able to revisit advice repeatedly, while mere verbal advice could be lost. She also found that texting encouraged self-expression and self–reflection in her clients as well as helping them in a crisis. It also helped her to assess her clients' mental state by their overall construction of the message. A meta-analysis by Head et al. (2013) on RCT studies in text messaging showed opportunities for improving a range of health outcomes. They found that text messaging is particularly effective when messages were tailored and personalized including tailoring the delivery schedule of the message. It was cost-effective and an effective intervention even without additional modalities. They also found that text messaging without a theory base was just as effective, contrary to some findings by Noar (2008) and others. However, they did accept that there could be methodological weaknesses in their meta-analysis.

Mobile phoning is an effective platform for health behaviour intervention. Technology-based intervention is a fast growing industry in health. 'Gamification' is a term used to describe the use of game design in a non-game context aim to motivate and improve user experience and engagement, taking responsibility for one's own health and promoting sustained behaviour change for good health, for example in the area of physical activity (Lister et al., 2014), chronic health management (Miller, Cafazzo and Seto, 2014), diabetes management (Boulos, 2015). Using rewards such as points, medals for feedback and encouragement, it focuses on user engagement and motivation. In a review of gamification in health and fitness apps, Lister et al. (2014) found that this early development lacked the integration of comprehensive behaviour theories which could have an impact on the efficacy of behaviour change; for example the ability of an individual to maintain and perform the behaviour. Further in-depth evaluation is needed to demonstrate its potential in health improvement. The input of clinicians and behavioural scientists is also essential in the delivery of effective intervention grounded in theoretical framework (King et al., 2013).

Social media as a setting for health promotion

The terms internet platform, internet environment, internet community are commonly used. Gold et al. (2012) used the term 'novel setting', others called it Virtual setting (Loss et al., 2013). 'Setting' is an interesting concept. Loss et al. (2013) consider the social network site as a setting and compared the use of social media space with the Setting Approach to health promotion, based on a range of definitions. They accept the social networking site as an attractive new setting, an important 'communicative social venue' for young people (Loss et al., 2013: 169). However, there is a lack of research and evaluation on its use based on the definition of setting approaches. Bennett and Glasgow (2009) agree that internet interventions have the potential for broad population reach; the currently limited evidence suggests that there are low levels of actual reach across a range of settings such as healthcare. They felt that the future of internet interventions lies in their dissemination potential. Since most definitions of 'setting' are based on the thinking of activities and the social, cultural and physical context of the environment in the late twentieth century, i.e. pre-Web 2.0 technologies in the twenty-first century, it is understandable that there is a cautious use of the term.

Further developments in modern technology and health promotion

Limited computer literacy limits the effective use of modern technologies. We also need to consider accessibility issues; people from low-income families who may not be able to afford the many modern digital devices or easy internet access; for example new wearable devices with health apps such as Fitbit and smartphone (Patel et al.,

2015); people with physical or other impairments who may have difficulties in accessing digital technologies; people with medical conditions such as epilepsy; 'technophobes'. Older people can also be seen as digital immigrants or 'digital visitors' in the use of digital technology (White and Le Cornu, 2011); many areas have poor internet connections . . . Miniwatts Marketing Group (2012) found limited use of the internet in some geographic areas of (e.g.) African countries, Middle East, Latin America and Asia. However, a study in Kenya showed that the use of short messaging services has increased the adherence of anti-retroviral treatment in HIV patients (Lester et al., 2010). Mobile technologies such as mobile phones are not only widely used in many developing countries. Our experience has been of mobile phones being very common among our health promotion students in African countries (Zambia, Ghana and The Gambia). We have also seen, when training African health promoters, the increased use of smartphones, tablets, iPads and dongles among many African health promoters. However, poor connectivity and the lack of (or unreliability of) an electricity supply can be challenging. Time and space are now no longer key limiting factors in knowledge-based decision-making. Good communication and connectivity are now basic requirements for information processing. Mobile communication technology reaches into every corner of the world. Health communicators need to be attentive to the possibility of communication inequalities (Koch-Weser, 2010). The future of internet interventions lies in their dissemination potential (Bennett and Glasgow, 2009).

Many health educators use a range of digital technologies and social media in their practice, although there are some 'laggards' (Hanson et al., 2011). Health promotion must engage with social media (Green et al., 2015). Many efficacy reports on internet interventions for public health issues have been encouraging (Bennett and Glasgow, 2009). However, research evaluation of the use of social media for health promotion is still limited (Loss et al., 2013), with internet usage in health interventions limited to traditional Web 1.0 channels. Further research on the importance and effectiveness of multiple methods of communication is required if health practitioners are to influence the levers and processes of health decision-making (Ratzan, 2011b). Use of these new initiatives also needs support from management, as well as careful planning to minimize any risks involved; for example, the exposure of unhealthy influences, equity issues relating to the access of technology and health literacy skills, cyber safety, while promoting physical activity and decreasing screen time among young people, as noted by the Centre for Health Promotion Women's and Children's Health Network (2012). Recommendations suggested for future development include the improvement of workforce skills, governance and leadership, the development of partnerships to support the use, planning and evaluation of social media strategies, developing workforce skills and ensuring resources to support its use. Gold et al. (2012) agreed that there is a need for health promotion intervention developers to understand more how social media can be used, how the internet is being used by the target audience and the need for adequate resources.

Implication for Practice 3

Do you use digital technology or social media for your health promotion work? What kind of resource and skills would you need in developing a health promotion campaign using these modern technologies? Has any evaluation been done on your electronic health promotion work?

Mass media, social change and empowerment

Mass communication media plays a powerful role in society. Mass media increasingly influences our attitudes, our identities, our consciousness (Berger, 2012). There is a danger of being mesmerized by all of the possibilities, especially in an innovative era, and of failing to be critical about the different types of change that are achievable. Change might not simply be about selecting the best technology but also about being critical about the intentions and purposes of the owners and controllers of this technology. We have already discussed the commercialization of mass media and the consumerist approach that the media often takes. A Marxist perspective would assert that the mass media is owned by the ruling class, that the media plays a key role in creating a sense of false consciousness in the working class, to promote capitalism and maintain a social, cultural and political hegemonic domination (Berger, 2012). However, reflecting our previous discussion, it is also important to note that even if there is a ruling-class-controlled mass media, it, too, does not have a magic bullet, as in Lasswell's formula. There is always 'noise' in the channel that distorts the message. Messages can also be filtered through other channels as described in the two-step model and Diffusion of Innovation (McQuail, 2010). If as health promoters we are seeking to bring about social changes, not merely at an individual (behavioural) level but also wider (societal and political) levels, we must explore issues of power and control as discussed in Chapter 2.

Health promotion seeks to bring about social change. We need to take into account the social context. Even without a Marxist perspective, it is important to be aware of the social and political limitations of health promotion in our comparatively consensual, orderly and well-informed society which is democratic, liberal and pluralistic (McQuail, 2010). Policy decisions and practice change reflect the societal, political and organizational values, the interests and views of those in positions of social, economic and political power. Media advocacy may have an important role to play, but policy changes take time. Policy development depends on who is involved in the policy-making process and on government ideology. We seek to enable people to be empowered to take action to bring about changes in their lives. Health promotion is about building agency in the individual and social capital in the community, in order to bring about changes – an asset-based approach. From a social reform perspective of education, the objective of education is collective/societal change, not simply individual change. Effective education seeks to change society. Learning is less about how knowledge is created, and more about by whom and for what purpose. Learners are taught about values and ideologies. They are encouraged and empowered to take social action to improve their lives (Pratt et al., 2005). See Chapter 3 on Educational Theory.

This leads on to debates on the use of persuasive messages to change behaviour as against empowerment of individual and communities. As discussed in Chapter 2 and Chapter 9, persuasive communication is a prominent feature in mass media communication. The use of persuasive power in mass media has been evident from the start. The powerful position of the media, the persuasiveness of health messages and how mass media is used are all too familiar, as seen in McGuire's communication/persuasion model (1989). There is no doubt that mass media communication can be powerful and effective. Health promotion is about empowerment. However, mass media is often a top-down approach, one-way communication. A public communication campaign's purpose is to inform, persuade, or motivate behaviour change in a relatively well-defined and large audience (Rice and Atkin, 2009). It can be used to inform a debate, as in media advocacy, but the strategic selection of information used can be manipulated to convince people. There is an agenda. The communicator shapes this. As we can see, for example, on television, the audience may well send e-mails, or comments on Twitter, but it is the producer or director who chooses who is being interviewed, which story is used, which comments are mentioned, what evidence is selected in the documentary. There are organizational constraints on what is to be released and what is not, where health promoters don't have control over the news channel's reporting (Green et al., 2015). Information can seem factual and authoritative. However, the credibility of information can be questionable and tailored to improve ratings and impact. It is the newsworthy items that receive more attention and get reported or even sensationalized to improve audience reach. A good health promotion message may not be headline grabbing.

Implication for Practice 4

Think about your role in reducing health inequalities and addressing social determinants of health. If health promotion is about social change, bringing about social justice, how can you as a health promoter address this in your day-to-day practice? What kind of communication methods would you use to achieve this?

Summary of key points

This chapter has provided a critical overview of methods and media in health communication. Specifically it has:

- discussed mass media communication in health and related theoretical perspectives such as Diffusion of Innovation
- considered the use of mass media for advocacy
- examined the evidence base for effectiveness of various methods of communication such as emotional appeal and peer education
- analysed the development of electronic and social media for communication such as the internet, the use of mobile phones and text messaging

Reflection 1 – How does mass media compare with interpersonal communication? Can mass media change behaviour?

Reflection 2 – Logical debate, news, documentary can seem factual, but how credible is the information? Do you believe information reported in the news or in documentary programmes?

Reflection 3 – Have you ever used shock tactics to get your clients to do what you want them to do? Is it ethical to frighten people? How effective, do you think, is the use of entertainment and celebrities in health promotion? Do people follow their iconic figures?

Reflection 4 – Do you use digital technologies in your practice? What are the issues and challenges that you have come across? How might you overcome them?

Further reading

Cross, R., O'Neil, I. and Dixey, R. (2013) Communicating health. In Dixey, R. (ed.) (2013) *Health Promotion: Global Principles and Practice.* Wallingford: CABI.
Chapter 4 'Communicating Health' is a very useful chapter, which gives a summary of and an insight into communication methods and communicating health messages.
Green, J., Tones, K., Cross, R. and Woodall, J. (2015) *Health Promotion: Planning and Strategies.* 3rd edn. London: Sage.
Chapter 7 'Education for Health' has many helpful insights. It looks at the communication process linking to education theories, persuasion and attitude change. It is a useful chapter to help you in considering different communication methods.
Wakefield, M. A., Loken, B. and Hornik, R. C. (2010) Use of mass media campaigns to change health behaviour. *Lancet,* 376, 1261–71.
This is a useful article in which the authors discuss the effectiveness and use of mass media as a communication method.

6

Social Marketing

Key aims

- To describe the key features of social marketing in relation to health communication and health promotion
- To examine the application of social marketing approaches to health communication and health promotion
- To explore international research on the use and effectiveness of social marketing to promote health
- To examine the challenges and contradictions of using social marketing as a means of promoting health

Introduction

This chapter will give an overview of social marketing, outline what it is and highlight how it can be applied to health communication and health promotion. It will review the literature on social marketing examining the relevance of it to health communication and establishing the strengths and limitations of social marketing as a strategy for health promotion. Taking a critical stance, this chapter will explore the efficacy of social marketing and will look at how social marketing has been utilized in a variety of international contexts. It will also examine the confusing and often competing relationship of social marketing as a strategy for promoting health. Links are made with other content in this book such as the discussion about the use of mass media methods in health communication in Chapter 5.

An overview of social marketing

There is a broad literature that describes what social marketing *is*. It is not the purpose of this chapter to provide a detailed exploration; for this, readers are directed elsewhere. Instead this chapter aims to consider social marketing as a means for health communication and promotion. To start with, however, this section will briefly describe the key features of social marketing as applied to health. For more detailed information the reader is invited to use the sources listed at the end of this chapter.

The case of social marketing in health communication and efforts to promote health is well established. Back in 1994 Buchanan et al. (1994: 56) commented that 'social marketing is here and its increased use seems inevitable'. We can attest that this certainly remains the case as we finalize this chapter content. It is important to note at the outset that social marketing approaches have been largely developed and applied in developed economic contexts (Carrete and Arroyo, 2014). Indeed, the American-centric nature of social marketing has also been highlighted by some such as Lindridge et al. (2013). This 'Western' bias is reflected in the wider research and literature on social marketing. A cursory glance at the literature reveals a plethora of research from the global north although, latterly, there is more work being published from 'emerging' economies. This is a highly salient point because, as McLeay and Olethorpe (2013: 232) point out, 'developing countries face quite different social issues and market environments'.

Advocates of social marketing for health are plentiful. French et al. (2010) argue that social marketing is an important tool for promoting public health while Hastings and Stead (2006) contend that social marketing can provide useful insights into how to influence human behaviour. Crawshaw and Newlove (2011: 136) describe social marketing strategies for health as adopting 'the methods of commercial marketing to promote social good through encouraging behavioural change in individuals'. In addition Campbell et al. (2014: 327) propose that it is 'an effective strategy for promoting healthy attitudes and influencing behaviours'. Social marketing has allure; after all, commercial marketing efforts are supremely successful. If they were not, then vast sums of money would not be poured into advertising.

In its broadest sense social marketing for health is about applying the principles of marketing to health drawing on techniques proven to promote commercial products (Evans and McCormack, 2008).

The principles of exchange, audience segmentation and competition are key to marketing.

Exchange is the first key principle under consideration. This is basically the idea that, in order to get something, you have to give something up. In short, there is some kind of cost involved. This principle is predicated on the idea of 'self-interest' – that people will take up something new, or change their behaviour if it is of benefit to them. Social marketing for health would emphasize social benefits such as better health and well-being (Green et al., 2015). Typically people will choose an outcome that has greater benefits, assuming, of course, that they aspire to having better health. There tends to be an emphasis on the voluntary nature of this (Lefebvre and Flora, 1988) although this notion is open to contention.

Social marketing puts the 'consumer' (or 'audience') at the centre of the process (Green et al., 2015). This second principle is referred to as *audience segmentation*. Its premise is that populations can be segmented or broken up into smaller units based on factors such as, for example, demographics, geography, socio-economic factors, lifestyle, personality and perceptions (Brocklehurst et al., 2012; Green et al., 2015). It is really important to understand your target audience in order to *create* 'need' or 'want'. As Carins and Rundle-Thiele (2013) argue, the assumption in marketing is that of *heterogeneity* – one size does not fit all. Brocklehurst et al. (2012) point out that different target audiences have different values and want different things. If you know your audience you are better placed to promote your 'product'.

The focus is on consumer *wants* and *needs* developing messages, solutions and products which are attractive to each group of people. This is described as *consumer orientation* (Donovan and Henley, 2010) – identifying and responding to the needs of the target audience; asking questions such as 'how are groups of people alike?', 'how do they differ?', 'why do they differ?' By doing so we can identify sub-groups or sub-populations of people based on values, aspirations and behaviours (Lynch et al., 2014). It is also necessary to understand what is competing for your target audience's time, effort and attention. In a tobacco awareness social marketing campaign in an Aboriginal community various local audiences were identified as requiring support. Messages were tailored to each different group of community members. The message for community members over 40 years of age was 'it's never too late' (to give up smoking); for young people 'smoking ain't cool no more' (in an effort to de-normalize a local culture of young adults smoking); and 'make our kids proud' which promoted a message presenting parents who have stopped smoking as 'heroes' for their children emphasizing the positive impacts of quitting on the whole family (Campbell et al., 2014: 340). Social marketing for health is therefore about selling ideas, attitudes or behaviours (Weinreich, 2006). Of course we are also faced with the timeless challenge that knowledge does not translate into behaviour change. The question is then how we 'market' behaviour change for health gain in an attractive and appealing way. Brocklehurst et al. (2012: 89) examined the role of social marketing in reducing oral health inequalities. They concluded that 'many questions remain [but] a greater knowledge of the behaviour of different subgroups of the population [or target audiences] and their reaction to health interventions would be a beneficial step'.

Geodemographics perhaps has something to offer here. Geodemographics is described as classifying people according to place (where they live) which 'says something about the characteristics of that person or group of people ... categorizing individuals into different types and groups of people according to similarities in their socio-economic circumstances, lifestyles and behavioural patterns' (Farr et al., 2008: 450). The usefulness of geodemographics to social marketing is clear and it has similarities with community mapping. The concept of audience segmentation is not unproblematic, however. Newton et al. (2013) point to the ethical difficulties of leaving some groups 'untargeted' while others benefit from a campaign. Presumably it is typical for those designing social marketing interventions to have a sound justification for focusing on certain sectors of the population and not others. Such decisions may be based on increased risk, higher levels of ill-health or inequalities of some kind. Newton et al. (2013) highlight the debate between consequentialist and non-consequentialist methods of audience segmentation in social marketing (based on cost-effectiveness and need respectively). They argue that either approach is ethical as long as it is well-justified and transparent. Newton et al. (2013: 1421) argue that 'in situations where there are known asymmetries in exposure to mass media channels, adopting a non-segmented mass-media approach may unintentionally entrench pre-existing disparities in health knowledge'. The implications are that a segmented or targeted approach is vital in order to address inequities.

Competition is the third and final principle in the social marketing approach. In social marketing the competition is, more often than not, existing behaviour and the benefits of it (Kotler et al., 2002). A literature review by Carins and Rundle-Theile (2013) concluded that *competitive analysis* was lacking in the majority of social marketing interventions. However, they argued that it is important to identify what is competing for the time, attention and effort of the audience. It is not easy for health promotion to compete against other 'forces'. Existing or current behaviour is often more attractive than changing. Likewise health communication must compete against other strong messages. For instance, Kapetanaki et al. (2014) highlight the negative impact that international food companies and retailers have on food choices promoting foods that are 'unhealthy' (high in sugar, fat and salt). Health communication messages are pitted against this. A better strategy might therefore be to work in partnership with such organizations in order to achieve 'greater social good' through improvements in health. Unfortunately in a capitalist, profit-driven context this is a difficult challenge.

In addition to the three principles of exchange, audience segmentation and competition the four 'Ps' of the marketing mix are also salient. These are 'product', 'price', 'promotion' and 'placement'. Each of these is now considered in turn.

In commercial marketing the *product* is key. Aschemann-Witzel et al. (2012: 146) describe the focus on general behaviours (in social marketing) as compared with a specific product (in commercial marketing) as a 'major conceptual difference' and contrast 'avoidance' (of unhealthy behaviours) with 'desire' (of an object). This highlights the complexity of 'the product' in social marketing where essentially it is behaviour or behavioural change (Kotler et al., 2002) but may in fact be 'a thing, an idea, a practice or a service' (Windahl et al., 2009: 124). Crucially, the product needs to be attractive and accessible (Green et al., 2015). It could be health itself, feeling healthier, a new behaviour or a measurable outcome such as lower blood pressure or weight loss. The challenge is how to make the 'product' attractive, particularly when it may only result in a long-term or relatively intangible benefit (Grier and Bryant, 2005). The question is, how can we create such products? Or, indeed, how do we make health itself a desirable outcome when, as Lewis et al. (2013) argue, health is not typically a strong motivation for many people. Much of human behaviour, particularly with regard to consumption, is motivated by immediate rather than delayed gratification (Brocklehurst et al., 2012). Conversely, many benefits to health are only felt in the long(er) term. Whatever the product, it has to have appeal. Several authors have suggested that health communication messages in social marketing should therefore emphasize outcomes such as pleasure, enjoyment, social gains (increased attractiveness etc.) and happiness/ well-being (Coveney and Bunton, 2003). Notably these are related to positive notions of health aligned to a more holistic, salutogenic social model of health rather than biomedical outcomes. In addition there is the issue of negative demand to contend with. Negative demand 'refers to the challenge social marketers face in marketing a product or service for which the target audience has a distaste or lack of excitement' (Rochlen and Hoyer, 2005: 687). Finally, it is important to note that sometimes there *is* a tangible product. For example, Pfeiffer (2004: 81) notes the extensive use of social marketing in the global south to promote 'condoms, other contraceptives, oral rehydration solution, mosquito nets, clean water kits, vitamins, antibiotics, and iodized salt'.

Price is also important. In commercial marketing the price is, more often than not, fiscal. The consumer parts with cash in order to receive a product or a service. In social marketing for health, we are ultimately marketing or selling the notion of health through behaviour change. It is therefore necessary to consider the real cost to the consumer and what a valued outcome ('product') would look like to them. Cost might also be psychological or social in nature (Green et al., 2015). The price or cost for making healthier choices or changing behaviour can vary substantially and is relatively subjective too. For example, with regard to engaging in physical activity the *cost* to the individual might be significant effort, physical discomfort or 'giving up' time to exercise. In addition, the benefits of changing behaviour have to be seen to outweigh the benefits of not changing. There are obvious links here to behavioural economics or 'the economics of health behaviour' which is a body of work about how and why people make decisions to adopt more healthy behaviours (Lefebvre, 1997: 111).

Promotion refers to the means by which a product is 'advertised'.

For example, how messages are designed/disseminated and what methods or activities are used in the process (Green et al., 2015). As Green et al. (2015) argue, this depends on understanding the other elements of the marketing mix, the audience and communication channels. Message framing is important here in establishing a product that is more desirable. Promotion therefore includes factors such as message design and distribution (Corcoran, 2013).

Placement refers to the location or positioning of the product. This includes where people might receive information as well as services (Green et al., 2015). Whatever the message or 'product', it has to be easily accessible and be positioned within a context where, for example, the behaviour takes place. Issues of convenience to the target audience also need to be taken into account here (Hubley and Copeman with Woodall, 2013).

Some advocate an additional 'p' – *Policy*. Policy is, of course, extremely important in the creation of supportive environments and facilitating change at a structural level. Policy is also important at the individual level. Brennan et al. (2010: 648) argue that, in policy terms, we need to 'develop initiatives that deliver personal, customized messages rather than generic communication initiatives'. In addition to policy Weinreich (2006) includes three further 'Ps' – 'Publics', 'Partnerships' and 'Purse-Strings'. *Publics* refers to the sectors of the population that the strategy is designed to address and links to target population and audience segmentation. *Partnerships* refers to engagement with partners who are central to ensure success of the strategy. Aschemann-Witzel et al. (2012) advocate that public-private partnerships should be formed in order to share expertise as well as partnering with advertising, communication and consumer behaviour experts. This is view espoused by Gesser-Edelsburg et al. (2014) who, in a study examining the importance of the role of opinion leaders in nutritional labelling in Israel, concluded that co-operation between different stakeholders was key. *Purse-strings* refers to whoever is funding the strategy; those who hold power in determining where efforts are directed.

Another important aspect of social marketing is the means by which messages are communicated. Decisions need to be taken as to what method to use to achieve the aim. This is dependent on a number of different factors such as the target audience and the 'product'. Mass media is often used in this process. The advantages and limitations of mass media approaches to promoting health are discussed in more detail in Chapter 5.

Green et al. (2015) argue that one of the key strengths of social marketing is that it provides a systematic planning process. The key stages of the process are the initial needs assessment (which is about knowing your audience), the implementation of the strategy and the evaluation of it. This has similarities with the process of health promotion planning.

Social marketing and theory

Social marketing may be described as a discipline (Lefebvre, 2013), process, framework or strategy but it is not a *theory* (Gordon et al., 2006). The effective application of social marketing in health promotion relies on a solid theoretical foundation (French and Blair-Stevens, 2006). Without such a foundation efforts are much more likely to be unsuccessful (Luca and Suggs, 2012). A range of theory may be drawn upon to underpin a social marketing approach including any theory that seeks to determine what influences behaviour and behaviour change. There is no right or wrong choice – it depends on what the overall aim and intended outcomes are. A range of different theories is commonly used – from social cognition theories to diffusion of innovations (see Chapters 4 and 5). For example, in a social marketing approach designed to increase walking Coulon et al. (2012) used an ecological framework to underpin the intervention.

Implication for Practice 2

Some reported social marketing programmes appear to lack reference to any relevant theoretical underpinning. Like any health communication or promotion programme, interventions using social marketing as an approach or strategy for health communication should be based on relevant and appropriate theory (for example, communication, education, behaviour change theory) in order to promote effectiveness.

The efficacy of social marketing approaches to promoting health – what is the evidence?

There is on-going debate about the effectiveness of social marketing approaches in promoting health. One might be forgiven for thinking that the increasing literature on this subject points to the fact that such approaches are successful; however, closer examination shows that this is not necessarily the case. Stead and Gordon (2010) noted that there is increasing pressure to produce evidence of effectiveness. In efforts to promote health this is an on-going and important concern more generally. A review by Carins and Rundle-Thiele (2013) examining thirty-four empirical studies concluded that a lot of interventions claiming to be based on social marketing are not actually using social marketing. Similarly when McDermott et al. (2005) carried out a review on social marketing and nutrition interventions they found that it was difficult to find interventions that they would define as social marketing.

A systematic review of social marketing by Stead et al. (2007) found significant effectiveness in the short term but no evidence for effectiveness in the medium and longer term. Nevertheless there does appear to be some evidence that social marketing is effective in changing health behaviours. Indeed, Evans and McCormack (2008) have argued that this evidence is substantial. However, a systematic review by Janssen et al. (2013) which sought to determine the effectiveness of social marketing strategies in changing alcohol-related attitudes and behaviour was inconclusive. The authors concluded that this was due to a number of reasons such as the different ways in which studies used social marketing principles, the different behavioural goals, whether or not the intervention was theory-based and the length of time that an intervention took. Of course, one of the difficulties in determining effectiveness is in constituting and/or measuring success. Typically there are no agreed benchmarks for this. As a means to establish whether social marketing was in fact being 'done' Andreasen (2002) proposed a framework which outlines six benchmarking criteria: (1) Behaviour Change, (2) Consumer Research, (3) Segmentation and Targeting, (4) Marketing Mix, (5) Exchange and (6) Competition. The UK National Social Marketing Centre (2010) has since added two more criteria – Theory and Customer Orientation.

Carins and Rundle-Thiele (2013) carried out a review of empirical work which reported the use of social marketing to address healthy eating. They noted, among other things, the lack of consistency across studies in terms of adopting social marketing benchmark criteria. Gordon et al. (2006) point out a number of other challenges including methodological limitations and the difficulties inherent in trying to isolate effect. Campbell et al.'s (2014) community-led social marketing campaign about tobacco used mixed methods to evaluate effect – surveys and interviews. The results indicated higher recall of messages associated with the campaign but notably 'intention to quit, and quit rates, was not evaluated' (Campbell et al., 2014: 340).

Research seems to suggest that there is 'reasonably strong evidence' (Gordon et al., 2006: 1139) that social marketing approaches are effective in nutrition interventions, less effective in smoking interventions and produce mixed results in interventions designed to address substance use or promote physical activity.

Evans and McCormack (2008) make several suggestions which may increase effectiveness including counter-marketing to counteract the effects of competing messages; providing credible and attractive arguments; using theory-based behaviour change models; using social modelling and behavioural alternatives and communicating 'risk' where the behavioural choices are clear. Other factors include promoting achievable, simple, clear behavioural outcomes (highlighting small steps to success); creating relevance; using multiple channels to disseminate the message and having an element of emotional engagement (Aschemann-Witzel et al., 2012). Different channels may be more successful with different audiences. As a result of their work on food storage times in the USA James et al. (2013) advocate using a mix of traditional and social media channels in order to increase the potential for intended behaviour change while Brennan et al. (2010) argue for the potential of new and emerging social media as mechanisms for spreading healthy-eating messages to young people. A substantial amount of work has been done using social marketing approaches to influence eating behaviours. Lessons from this body of work might be applicable to other public health concerns.

We turn now to some global literature on social marketing in health and what appears to work, in what context and under what circumstances. The literature on social marketing has increased substantially over the past couple of decades. In the UK health policy has developed such that social marketing approaches form a central plank underpinning initiatives to tackle problems such as childhood and adult obesity. A cursory glance at the academic literature shows that social marketing approaches have been applied to a range of public health issues internationally. For example, promoting healthy eating in Greece (Kapetanaki et al., 2014), physical activity in African American populations (Coulon et al., 2012), increasing the use of insecticide treated bed nets (ITNs) in rural Tanzania (Schellenberg et al., 2001), promoting the uptake of injectable contraceptives in Ethiopia (Prata et al., 2011) and examining unhealthy food choices in Nigeria (McLeay and Oglethorpe, 2013).

Aschemann-Witzel et al. (2012) outline lessons learned from commercial food marketing which they argue can be applied to shaping healthier food choice behaviour. They concluded that 'whether or not a particular factor contributes to future success depends on the specific context of the use, the combinations of factors and the environment' (p. 139). Similarly Lindridge et al. (2013) argue that economic, environmental and social influences should be taken into account. Research by Logie-MacIver and Piacentini (2011) points to the important role of social context in long-term behaviour change. Likewise Lynch et al. (2014) highlight the importance of other people and their influence on health behaviours in terms of providing support.

In a study by Kapetanaki et al. (2014) that examined the use of social marketing to promote healthier eating in a student population in Greece, the barriers to healthier food choices were noted to be lack of time, fast-food availability and taste, peer pressure, lack of knowledge and lack of family support. Conversely healthier eating was motivated by good health, appearance and psychological consequences. Notably the lack of supportive environments was a key factor in less healthy food choices. There is a clear link to the five action areas of the Ottawa Charter (World Health Organization, 1986) here and the role of policy and environment in promoting food choice. Kapetanaki et al. (2014) note the failure of food policy to support healthier food choices for students in tertiary education within the Grecian context. This then puts the responsibility for health firmly with the individual – to make the healthiest choices within an environment that competes heavily to promote unhealthy choices. Kapetanaki et al. (2014) therefore argue that social marketing approaches to promoting healthier choices should take place alongside efforts to effect change at structural levels such as increasing the availability of healthier foods and lowering prices.

A study in the USA by Martinez Donate et al. (2010) points to the effectiveness of a social marketing campaign for increasing condom use and HIV testing in heterosexually identified Latino men who have sex with men and women, yet it also concludes that more research is needed. In terms of effectiveness, in Mexico a social marketing campaign was used to promote Mexico City's 2008 comprehensive smoke-free law. A paper assessing the impact of this campaign concluded that 'social marketing campaigns can reinforce knowledge and attitudes that favour smoke-free laws, thereby helping to establish smoke-free norms' (Thrasher et al., 2011: 328). In the context of myth-busting in Pakistan Qureshi and Shaikh (2006) argue that social marketing might be an effective way to motivate behaviour change. They cite a specific example of a successful social marketing campaign in Pakistan that increased the use of iodized salt. It reportedly 'produced impressive results in a short period of time' (p. 136). There is some evidence that combining social marketing strategics with community-based distribution of certain types of 'product' such as injectable contraceptives (Prata et al., 2011) or ITNs (Schellenberg et al., 2001) is more effective. Such approaches take advantage of existing community networks sometimes compensating community members with a small portion of the proceeds from sales by way of incentive.

> ### Implication for Practice 3
>
> Interventions using social marketing as an approach or strategy for health communication must clearly define key terms and have built-in means of evaluation from the outset in order to determine effectiveness. Equally, well-defined outcomes (whether immediate, short-term or long-term in nature) are important for assessing success.

Social marketing and health promotion – uneasy bedfellows?

Behaviour and behaviour change is complex. Different factors interact to produce behavioural responses. As discussed in Chapter 4 mainstream behaviour change theories have fallen short for a number of different reasons and are therefore open to critique. The complexity of behaviour and behavioural choices presents a challenge to social marketing approaches as much as any other approach to promoting health. It is this complexity which some would argue has hindered efforts and curtailed positive outcomes. The question remains, if the evidence of effectiveness is somewhat limited why do we continue to put resources into such approaches – particularly the more 'downstream' efforts at an individual level?

Although over twenty years ago, Buchanan et al. (1994: 49) raised concerns about the 'limits of social marketing and [the] potential iatrogenic side-effects of using social marketing strategies' to promote health, it is argued by Green et al. (2015) that health promotion and social marketing have commonalities. They are optimistic about the potential for social marketing to address health inequalities and tackle the social determinants of health. They point to the UK National Social Marketing Centre's (2007) efforts at understanding the wider context in which people make behavioural choices and the focus on policy/strategy level. Nevertheless they voice caution with regard to differences in emphases and values (Green et al., 2015).

Note, for example, the apparent contradictions between a focus on behaviour change and an empowerment stance and the creation of supportive environments versus the emphasis on individual change. Nevertheless, Griffiths et al. (2008) presented a strong case for health promotion and social marketing to work together for health improvement arguing that this was the most likely route to success.

There appears to be a disconnect between the way in which social marketing is applied to health and the rhetoric of social marketing in terms of addressing social problems and creating social good at a population level. These claims are undermined by the focus on individual behaviour change. Although some might argue that greater social good can be achieved by change at this level (after all, populations are made up of individuals), the ethos of health promotion would suggest otherwise. Focusing on individual behaviour change inevitably leads to victim-blaming, a position which does not sit at all well with notions of empowerment. Crawshaw and Newlove (2011: 138) take up this position and offer a rather damning report – 'social marketing for health, although ostensibly intended to bring about "social good", rather, eschews the social in favour of an individualization of responsibility for the management of the body, health and self'.

In the UK and other contexts such as the USA, the governance of health has been devolved to the level of the individual. The use of social marketing approaches in public health and health promotion efforts reinforces this political agenda (French et al., 2009). The pursuit of health within a neoliberal context (health citizenship) firmly locates health as both the property and responsibility of the individual (Crawshaw and Newlove, 2011) – see Chapter 9 for further discussion on these issues.

'Upstream' social marketing

One of the key criticisms of social marketing is its 'downstream' focus on behavioural actions and practices rather than on the more 'upstream' focus on structural determinants of health that characterizes health promotion (Brocklehurst et al., 2012; Pfeiffer, 2004). We can distinguish between *downstream* and *upstream* social marketing. Gordon (2013: 15–25) differentiates between the two as follows: 'downstream social marketing focuses on behaviour change at the individual level while upstream social marketing focuses on behaviour change at policy-maker level', i.e. in terms of influencing structural factors and the environment(s) in which behaviour at an individual level occurs. This is an important distinction. Clearly the more upstream efforts are the more closely they are aligned with the underpinning philosophical foundations of health promotion which seek to move attention away from the individual level towards the wider determinants of health. Coulon et al. (2012) carried out a study using a social marketing approach to promote physical activity among African Americans. The results appeared positive indicating that the participants not only reported walking more but also better social connectedness. However, a number of 'upstream' factors influenced the participants' levels of engagement in physical activity such as a lack of safe places to be active and lack of community support. In addition, the participants were described as being part of an 'underserved' African American community '(low-income, high-crime)' (Coulon et al., 2012). The authors do acknowledge that environmental and ecological factors were significant in causing structural barriers to community-walking such that off-duty police and county officials were hired to control stray dogs and ensure walker safety (Coulon et al., 2012). Nevertheless this illustrates the importance of tackling upstream determinants. Critics of social marketing, Crawshaw and Newlove (2011: 138), argue that social marketing efforts are not able to address upstream concerns stating that while they 'attempt to promote change in the contexts in which health behaviours take place, they are unable to address wider structural factors which both determine and inhibit behaviour at a local level'. There are those, however, who are more optimistic about potential synergies such as Dibb and Carrigan (2013: 1384) who argue that social marketing 'requires the development of an integrated approach addressing both upstream and downstream stakeholders simultaneously' advocating joined-up rather than fragmented approaches.

Gordon et al. (2006: 1133) maintain that social marketing has potential for improving health at structural levels. In their review of social marketing interventions they concluded that 'there is evidence that social marketing interventions can work with a range of target groups, in different settings, and can work upstream as well as with individuals'. This point was reiterated by Carins and Rundle-Thiele (2013: 1636) who argued that 'consideration must be given to the changes that can be made to social and environmental influences on behaviour'.

The box below shows a worked example of downstream versus upstream social marketing interventions in promoting physical activity whereby the two different approaches are applied to the issue.

This example illustrates the contrast between the more individualistic and reductionist focus of downstream approaches in social marketing and the much broader scope of upstream approaches.

'Downstream' versus 'Upstream' Social Marketing intervention: A worked example on promoting Physical Activity

Downstream

- Promote positive attitudes to physical activity
- Encourage individuals to change their behaviour i.e. take up cycling; walk more

Upstream

- Governmental departments responsible for the built environment and transport to increase structural opportunities for safer cycling and walking i.e. dedicated cycle lanes; 'green' spaces; safer places to walk and run
- Policy level initiatives promoting cycle/walk to school/work schemes
- Employers and institutions subsidizing the cost of bicycles and cycling equipment/establishing walking groups

Implication for Practice 4

Recognizing and being aware of competing interests and issues of power is critical in appraising any evidence of effectiveness of social marketing approaches to promoting health. Upstream approaches to social marketing fit well with a more critical approach to health communication and are instrumental in addressing the wider social determinants of health.

Challenges and criticisms

Up until this point in the chapter we have resisted providing definitions of social marketing for health. However, to further develop our critique it is now prudent to do so. Three definitions are presented and discussed.

1 Weinreich (2006) defines social marketing as 'the application of commercial marketing technologies to ... programmes designed to influence the voluntary behaviour of target audiences' and Smith (undated) as 'the use of marketing principles to influence a

target audience (individual group or society) to voluntarily accept, reject, modify or abandon a behaviour' (see www.aed.org). Note the similarities with regard to the use of the word 'voluntary'. On the surface this implies notions of freedom of choice leaving it up to the individual to make a choice about whether or not they change their behaviour. Individualistic, deterministic and neoliberal discourse is, however, inherent within such definitions.

2 The Department of Health (2008a) defines social marketing as 'the systematic application of marketing concepts and technique to achieve specific behavioural goals relevant to a social good'. This definition calls into question the utilitarian concept of 'social good' challenging the theoretical leap from change at an individual level to outcomes of benefit at population level. One might reasonably question 'whose good?', 'to what end?' and 'who serves to gain?'.

3 French and Blair-Stevens (2006: 2) define social marketing as 'the systematic application of marketing concepts and techniques to achieve specific behavioural goals to improve health and to reduce health inequalities'. This definition appears more in line with the social concerns at the heart of health promotion philosophy and efforts, yet it is not clear how the achievement of behavioural goals at an individual level will have a direct impact on wider health inequalities. On the contrary, we know that in order to have an effect significant change is required at structural levels such as policy and economics. Indeed, as Kapetanaki et al. (2014: 176) succinctly argue, 'social marketing can only work effectively when combined with other initiatives like education, policies, regulations and advocacy and should never be considered separately from the wider, integrated context of [health promotion] initiatives and policies'.

There are several generic challenges and critiques that can be levelled at social marketing for health. Many of them relate to issues in health communication more generally as discussed throughout this text. Evans and McCormack (2008) highlight message-clutter as an issue. In a world where information is readily available at our fingertips the sheer volume of it can be overwhelming. In addition, much of it may be complex and contradictory.

In summary Grier and Bryant (2005) outline four categories of challenge for the use of social marketing in public health: (1) misconceptions and other barriers to diffusion; (2) formative research and evaluation methodologies; (3) theoretical issues; and (4) ethical considerations. For a more detailed discussion, see Grier and Bryant's

(2005) paper *'Social Marketing in Public Health'*. Despite these challenges, however, Grier and Bryant (2005) advocate the use of social marketing approaches in efforts to promote public health. Specifically they outline the value of community involvement championing the direct participation of 'consumers as partners in the planning process' (p. 336). However, Pfeiffer (2004) points out the relative exclusion of communities in social marketing approaches to health promotion. An exception to this is the social marketing campaign around tobacco control in Aboriginal communities in New South Wales referred to earlier in this chapter (Campbell et al., 2014). Campbell et al. (2014) outline the development, implementation and evaluation of Kick the Habit Phase 2 which is a locally based strategy that included community members in the design and delivery of the campaign described as 'a smoking cessation social marketing campaign *by and for* Aboriginal communities' (p. 328, our emphasis). The paper also raises the important question of whether mainstream health communication campaigns are appropriate for use with indigenous groups suggesting that they may not be as effective.

In relation to condom social marketing in Mozambique Pfeiffer (2004) highlights the importance of community involvement. He outlines the difficulties involved in trying to promote condom use in avoiding HIV within a context where Pentecostal and African Independent Churches promote contrary (anti-condom) messages about sexuality and risk behaviours, namely 'fidelity and the sanctity of family' (p. 79). In addition Pfeiffer (2004) notes the recourse to sex work that is necessary for the survival of those living in poverty. Such structural issues form the backdrop to any social marketing campaign. Pfeiffer (2004) offers a compelling argument – 'this clash of messages illustrates how [social marketing] approaches to changing behaviours as complex and socially volatile as sexuality may not only be ineffective, but harmful because genuine community participation, dialogue, and monitoring are excluded from the process, while structural determinants and social context of "high-risk" behaviour are left unaddressed' (p. 79). This point was reiterated in a later social marketing campaign to promote protected sexual practices in Cuba. Cultural resistance and deep rooted stigma about condom use proved to be a significant challenge (Nery Suárez Lugo, 2013).

Australian authors Gurrieri et al. (2013: 128) specifically critique social marketing campaigns aimed at women and are scathing in their attack on 'government-defined agenda of "healthism"'. They argue that social marketing reinforces bodies as sites of control, promotes the neoliberal notion of 'body as project' and is driven by 'consumption-based individualism' (Gurrieri et al., 2013: 129). This, in turn, minimizes women's lived experiences and can promote stigma and victim-blaming. The Change for Life campaign in England is a case in point. Designed to address childhood obesity the campaign reflects a government-led agenda and is funded by the Department of Health. Closer examination of the campaign reveals explicit regulatory discourse whereby those targeted are exhorted to change behaviour and comply with expert-led advice around eating and physical activity.

There is an inherent ethical dilemma in social marketing for health, not least the conflict between personal freedom and the rights of the individual to behave in an autonomous way versus the 'greater good' agenda. This reflects the on-going political and moral debates around state and individual responsibility for health. There is also the tension between the use of health communication methods that appear to be more persuasive or coercive and methods that empower. Lastly, there is the question of which theory to use. We noted earlier the plethora of theoretical possibilities. The challenge then becomes about which theory to select to underpin the approach taken or the methods used. In addition there is a need to decide the best way of delivering the message, again theoretical considerations have value here.

Summary of key points

This chapter has provided a critical overview of social marketing and its use in health communication. Specifically it has:

- outlined the key features of social marketing in relation to health communication
- examined the application of social marketing approaches to health communication
- explored international research on the use and the effectiveness of social marketing in promoting health
- examined the challenges and contradictions of using social marketing as a means to promote health

Reflection 1 – Compare and contrast the key ideas in social marketing (features and approaches) and health promotion (principles and ethos). Can you identify any synergies and/or contradictions between the two? You may wish to then refer to the following debate paper: Griffiths, J.,

Blair-Stevens, C. and Thorpe, A. (2008) *Social marketing for health and specialized health promotion: Stronger together – weaker apart.* NSMC, Royal Society for Public Health. What do you think? Are health promotion and social marketing stronger together, weaker apart or would you take up another position? Try to justify what you think.

Reflection 2 – Following on from Reflection 1 consider again the relationship between social marketing and health promotion. Are there any differences or contradictions between the two sets of ideas? What might these mean for practice? Refer back to the paper by Griffiths et al. (2008). What practical and ethical tensions exist for those working in health communication and health promotion?

Reflection 3 – Find two papers within the peer-reviewed academic literature that use social marketing for the purposes of health communication. Compare and contrast the two. To what extent do the papers illustrate the difficulties and challenges that have been discussed in this chapter with regard to consistency of approaches in social marketing and challenges in establishing effectiveness? How might such challenges be addressed? What does the evidence base tell us about what works?

Reflection 4 – Select a health promotion/public health issue that interests you. How might a social marketing strategy be applied to that issue in order to effect positive behaviour change? What challenges might be encountered? What are the ethical implications? Compare and contrast upstream and downstream approaches. Which do you think would be most effective and why?

Further reading

French, J. and Gordon, R. (2015) *Strategic Social Marketing.* London: Sage. This is also available as an ebook.
This book provides useful detail on the theory and practice of social marketing as applied to social problems in areas including health, environment, governance and social policy drawing on a range of international examples. It is accompanied by a useful website.
Lefebvre, R. C. (2013) *Social Marketing and Social Change: Strategies and Tools for Health, Well-Being and the Environment.* San Francisco, CA: Jossey-Bass. This is also available as an online resource book.
This book is written by an expert in social marketing. It uses case studies and

research about social marketing to explain, in detail, what it is about and how it can be used to address complex problems.

Douglas Evans, W. and Hastings, G. (2008) *Public Health Branding: Applying Marketing for Social Change.* Oxford: Oxford University Press.

This text sets out an argument for the importance of public health branding as a critical strategy in changing population behaviours and achieving lasting health outcome benefits.

Social Marketing Quarterly – journal published by Sage.

This is a quarterly peer-reviewed international journal that publishes papers on the theory, research and practice of social marketing which is useful to both practitioners and scholars.

7

Health Literacy

Key aims

- to give a historical overview of the evolving concept of health literacy
- to locate the functionalist origins of functional health literacy
- to discuss the rise of functional health literacy
- to evaluate the suitability of functional health literacy to the radical agenda in health promotion
- to consider the use of key concepts and theories in health promotion to support the development of critical health literacy

Introduction

This chapter explores the concept of health literacy and its contribution to health communication in health promotion. We will outline a number of competing definitions that have emerged over the last twenty years and examine why, despite its continuing evolution, a functional understanding of health literacy predominates in English-speaking nations. Taking a critical historical perspective, we locate the origins of this functionalist orientation in the adult basic skills agenda of the 1990s which, advanced by the Organization for Economic Co-operation and Development (OECD), led to the development of the International Adult Literacy Survey (IALS) and mass adult literacy testing across North America and Western Europe. Based on IALS findings, low literacy became associated with poor levels of productivity, poor levels of economic growth and competitiveness. We identify a similar logic at work within functional health literacy

(FHL), where low literacy skills appear to correlate with poor health outcomes, resulting in burdensome costs to both state and society. In this chapter we will deconstruct these assumptions and critique the claims and limitations of FHL, and in turn we will present a critical conceptualization of health literacy for the radical health promotion practitioner to consider.

Overview of the evolving concept of health literacy

Health literacy may be defined as, 'the cognitive and social skills which determine the motivation and ability of individuals to gain access to, understand, and use information in ways which promote and maintain good health' (Nutbeam, 2000: 10). The need for these skills has grown in recent years, in tandem with neoliberal governments which encourage its citizens to take on more individual responsibility for their health. As a result, health literacy has become a key consideration in health communication, but it is not a new concept (Nutbeam, 2000; Ratzan, 2011b; Tones, 2002; Mackie, 2012). According to Ratzan (2011b) the term 'health literacy' was first used by Simonds in 1974 who made a case for health education to be taught in schools, so students might be as 'literate' in the subject of health as in other subjects from the taught curriculum. By the millennium health literacy had acquired a more technical meaning (Tones, 2002), focusing specifically on functional literacy and numeracy skills in order to facilitate an improved comprehension of health literature, advice and treatment, and also patient compliance (Murtha, 2015). The work of Nutbeam (1998, 2000) was extremely influential at this time, articulating to health communicators three distinct modes of health literacy practice: the functional, the inter-active and the critical mode. Functional Health Literacy (FHL) requires a level of basic skills in reading and writing to be able to function effectively in everyday situations, whereas Inter-active (or communicative) Health Literacy (IHL) requires more advanced cognitive and literacy skills that can be used to participate in everyday activities, as well as apply new information to changing circumstances. Critical Health Literacy (CHL) demands even more advanced cognitive skills which, together with social skills, can be applied to analyse information and to use this information to exert greater control over life events and situations.

Throughout the early years of the millennium continuous theorizing saw the concept of health literacy expand beyond Nutbeam's three modes of health literacy (1999) to include specific domains such as *scientific literacy* – the ability to understand scientific and medical concepts; *civic literacy* – the ability to design sound public health messages that encourage individual health literacy; and *cultural literacy* – which involves tailoring communication content to specific cultural groups (Zarcadoolas et al., 2005). Further expansion of the concept made way for *e-literacy* (Robinson and Robertson, 2010; Berry, 2007; Norman and Skinner, 2006) – a domain comprising information, computer and media skills reflecting the latest innovations in global communications and technology. Definitions of health literacy continue to evolve today (Rudd, 2015; Nutbeam, 2008), but we consider the latest UK trend towards multiple definitions problematic (mental and physical health literacy; sexual health literacy; health literacy for people with intellectual disabilities) with the potential to further confuse and render the concept of health literacy meaningless. Yet, despite this activity – and repeated calls for health literacy to become more critical (Sykes et al., 2013; Rowlands, 2012) and involve whole communities (WHO, 2009; Nutbeam, 2008; Kickbusch, 2001) – health literacy in practice has remained stubbornly functionalist, privileging a 'clinical' approach in health promotion which aims for better communication between healthcare professionals and patients in order to increase compliancy (Cuban, 2006; Pleasant and Kuruvilla, 2008).

Implication for Practice 1

What implications do these competing definitions of health literacy have for health communication and health promotion practice? What are the individual and organizational resource implications of each?

The origins of functional health literacy

To understand why health literacy is largely (but not exclusively) functionalist, we need to look to North America and to the field of adult basic education (ABE) where a number of studies emerged during the 1980s and early 1990s to suggest significant percentages of adults lacked the *general* literacy skills needed to function in everyday life (Kirsch, Jungeblut, Jenkins and Kolstad, 1993; Kirsch, Jungeblut and Campbell, 1992; Statistics Canada, 1991; Kirsch and Mosenthal, 1990; Kirsch and Jungeblut, 1986). From this research the OECD concluded, 'low literacy levels were a serious threat to economic performance and social cohesion' (OECD, 1992) prompting the first International Adult Literacy Survey (IALS) of 1994. From an initial membership of nine countries in 1994 (Canada, the USA, France, Germany, Ireland, the Netherlands, Poland, Sweden and Switzerland), an additional five joined in the second round in 1996 to include Australia, Great Britain, New Zealand and Northern Ireland, with a further nine countries participating in 1998 (Chile, the Czech Republic, Denmark, Finland, Hungary, Italy, Norway, Slovenia and the Italian-speaking region of Switzerland). Its purpose was to understand, 'the level and distribution of literacy within their adult populations, and [to] learn what can be done to improve literacy' because it was argued, 'adult literacy has come to be seen as crucial to the economic performance of industrialized nations' (Statistics Canada, 2005).

With the exception of Denmark, Finland, Germany, Netherlands, Norway and Sweden (Statistics Canada, 2000, p. xiii), IALS confirmed the original hypotheses of the early North American studies and substantiated the OECD's fears, revealing that – on average – at least one quarter of the adult population of working age lacked the basic literacy and numeracy skills deemed to be 'functional' in an industrialized economy (Statistics Canada, 2000). According to the levels developed by IALS, 'functionality' is described as a *level two* skill, which denotes the ability to identify words and numbers in context and to be able to respond with simple information, e.g. to be able to fill in a form. Level *three* reflects the skills generally expected upon completing high school/secondary school, for example, the ability to identify, understand, synthesize and respond to information. Level *five* is the highest level and represents a range of sophisticated skills which include being able to understand and verify the sufficiency of information as well as synthesize, interpret, analyse and discuss the information (Statistics Canada, 2005).

The findings from the first international survey (IALS, 1997) and indeed some of the national reports that followed – for example 'A Fresh Start' (UK) – presented an individualistic narrative that linked educational failure with economic and social exclusion. Further, it was claimed rather than *evidenced,* poor levels of performance at work impacted negatively on the nation's productivity and threatened to undermine international competitiveness (DfEE, 1999). Scant attention was paid to the true social costs of poor basic skills to individuals (whether in or out of work) or their effect on families and communities, or indeed upon society as a whole. In short, these reports completely failed to address poor literacy and numeracy in its rightful context: alongside (and sometimes a consequence of) other forms of social and economic disadvantage (Marmot, 2010, 2006). Over the course of a decade this came to dominate not only the discourses of education and the economy, but health also.

Implication for Practice 2

How does the discourse of individual deficit affect health promotion and health communication? Can lay perspectives be privileged effectively using a deficit approach?

In the same way literacy and numeracy levels were thought to mediate economic performance, so too did health. Poor levels of functional literacy led to low levels of health literacy, or so the argument went (Marshall, 2012) ultimately manifesting persistent symptoms of ill-health. Data available from the OECD nations seemed to support this view, revealing that those with the poorest educational attainment also had the poorest health (ONS, UK; Statistics Canada; Australian Bureau of Statistics; USA.gov; CSO Ireland). In a healthcare setting, this meant that if a quarter of all adults among the five major English-speaking nations had reading skills below level 2 (as IALS claimed), they would not be able to understand the general healthcare literature in circulation, or comprehend and follow important instructions for treatment. The immediate consequence of this would be increased hospital admissions, a rise in the inappropriate use or misuse of services such as the accident and emergency service and ultimately, a general rise in the mismanagement of long-term conditions (Davis, 2009).

According to the dominant neoliberal discourse this was a growing burden that the wealthiest nations on Earth could ill afford; and it is against this backdrop that two functionalist responses emerged which essentially involved (a) raising the general standard of adult literacy among the population and (b) simplifying written materials for the public (Balatti et al., 2009). This approach was taken up across all English-speaking industrialized nations – with North America leading the way. In the UK and Ireland governments addressed the so-called adult skills deficit by launching country-wide basic skills campaigns which focused on literacy, numeracy and English as a Second /Other Language (ESOL). In the UK, a contextualized basic skills course for healthcare was developed (Skilled for Health) which targeted both service users and employees without a level 2 qualification. Unsupported by government strategy or public funds, simplifying materials assumed a rather ad-hoc development – dependent upon expert knowledge and resources within organizations to screen existing materials and reproduce them in an easy-to-read format. We now look at these two strategies in turn to critique, in greater detail, the relevance of each strategy to health communication and health promotion.

Readability and the implications for health communication

Readability is an important attribute of written material and can affect the reader's ability to comprehend important messages (Badarudeen and Sabharwal, 2010). As the majority of health communication still relies on written material (leaflets; pharmaceutical information; dosages) it is vital that the message is accessible. According to Rudd, 'health materials are written at levels that exceed the average reading skills of the public' (2015: 7). Screening written materials using a manual readability test, e.g. SMOG (Simple Measure Of Gobbledegook) or using computer software programmes such as the Flesch–Kincaid test can help practitioners understand the level of clarity or complexity of a text. For a potential readership with low literacy skills a readability score of twelve is recommended, but this is quite challenging to achieve. (It should be noted that a readability score is the result of a quantitative test to measure *textual complexity*, not communicate arbitrary ideas about a person's 'reading age').

In terms of producing accessible written materials specialist skills are required to ensure that unnecessarily long and difficult words, professional jargon, poor punctuation and ill-thought-out sentences are avoided. Due to the widespread popularity of readability in recent years, across all sectors, a demand for these skills has grown and many organizations now commission or produce their own easy-to-read materials. The Harvard School of Public Health in the USA and the National Adult Literacy Agency (NALA) and Health Service Eire (HSE) in Ireland are particularly active in this area, championing the use of plain English in healthcare settings to promote greater health literacy (Rudd, 2015; Marshall, 2012). The demand has prompted an array of textbooks on the market and in-house toolkits to assist professionals address what Rudd calls 'the serious mismatch' between health information and the communication skills of the public (Rudd, 2012, 2015). Readability represents a cost-effective, pragmatic solution that has the potential to benefit almost everyone, augmenting written forms of communication with iconic and symbolic codes (Green et al., 2015) to better facilitate the comprehension of healthcare messages. Moreover, there are some noteworthy spin-offs with readability because the process exposes unnecessary value-laden statements (common in healthcare literature) resulting in user-friendly materials which do not draw attention to an individual's poor *reading* skills, but rather to the poor *writing* skills of the author!

Implication for Practice 3

What implications for health communication does the readability agenda have? In what ways could health promotion practitioners communicate more inclusively and effectively with the public? What role should written materials be given in communicating health?

On the surface, there appears to be a lot of common sense with the readability agenda improving the clarity of information facilitates comprehension, which in turn influences the decision-making process leading ultimately to changes in behaviour which, it is anticipated, comply with professional healthcare discourse. For the reasons that are discussed throughout this book, and because of the pernicious and continuing influence of the wider determinants of health, we know this to be false. Vulnerable communities that bear the greatest burden of ill-health have proved resistant in this respect (Rowlands, 2012; Department of Health, 2008b). But there is also this to consider: how likely is it that a person with poor literacy will read leaflets in order to gain information? Due to reasons of culture and habit, we suggest it is highly unlikely. As Parker and Guzmararian (2003) highlight, those in greatest need often have the poorest ability to understand health information and so it is probable that they have developed other ways and means of sourcing information, for example from friends and family, TV documentaries and soaps, the arts and other media such as radio, social media and the internet. Even close proximity to, and familiarity with healthcare services might be an effective experiential form of acquiring information and education.

The problem with this, if it is a problem, is that these informal methods of acquiring information and knowledge are difficult to measure and therefore difficult to gain evidence for (Peerson and Saunders, 2009). The importance of this in health promotion today cannot be underestimated for as Raphael writes, 'the issue of evidence has . . . become prominent in these times of economic rationalism as health promoters are increasingly asked to justify their activities by providing evidence of effectiveness' (Raphael, 2000). This is certainly an issue where outcomes-based frameworks have been adopted to measure the efficacy of health promotion interventions in public health (see Chapter 9). That said, measuring the contribution of traditional literacies (numeracy and literacy) to health literacy might soon be defunct in any case as technological advances are revolutionizing the way we communicate (Ratzan, 2011b), arguably replacing the need to be functional in English and maths. Modern life in the West has become very high-speed, globally connected, technology-rich, information-oriented and mobile which is reflected in the ubiquitous rise of the smartphone: mini personal computers storing huge amounts of data, capable of capturing, adapting and sharing data in a multiplicity of ways, instantly and globally, for further re-use. The nature and speed of these developments is truly global, with evidence of increased access and use of these devices in places of absolute poverty such as sub-Saharan Africa (Smith, 2014; Evans, 2012).

The impact of technology and globalization on communication is discussed in detail elsewhere in this volume, but in terms of FHL and the readability agenda a definitive shift has already occurred, marking the end of traditional literacies as a popular and necessary form of communication in favour of new digital literacies that are economical with language, and which replace the need for the three Rs with icons, audio-visuals, voice recognition and artificial intelligence (Ratzan, 2011c). The smartphone, with increasingly elaborate and sophisticated applications, is arguably the most accessible and inclusive means of communication in the twenty-first century. Yet, despite the booming growth in technology and 'apps' professional health organizations have been surprisingly slow to respond – particularly in public health where the focus has largely been on introducing technology to share and manage patient data (NHS Five Year Forward View, 2014).

Improving literacy and its contribution to functional health literacy

As we have highlighted, readability is a popular aspect of FHL, but this wasn't always so and clinicians who often produced public health information initially protested against an agenda which threatened to 'dumb-down' important messages. However, many professionals might have then been genuinely unaware just how much of the population was affected by low levels of literacy and numeracy, or indeed what 'low' actually meant (see www.nationalnumeracy.org.uk/what-do-levels-mean). Following high profile basic skills campaigns in the early years of the millennium, the repeated rounds of IALS and now the OECD's regular Programme for the International Assessment of Adult Competencies (PIAAC) this is arguably no longer the case. That said, a recent survey in Ireland showed only 31 per cent of GPs to be aware of the extent of low literacy in the Irish population (GP Omnibus Survey, 2009, cited in Marshall, 2012). Despite the relative success of readability Hoffman and McKenna (2006) believe much more could still be done if health promoters used readability to educate the public by stealth, or as Daghio et al. (2006) suggest, if practitioners involved lay people in the co-production of public literature. To realize such objectives in a sensitive manner would require a closer union between allied healthcare professionals (AHP) and educators – which is exactly what happened in the UK with the creation of contextualized basic skills courses at the turn of the last century (Skilled for Health) to which we now turn.

Before we comment on the efficacy of the educative approach to health literacy it is important to note a specific development that reorganized (and re-professionalized) the teaching and learning of basic skills, a development which privileged a functionalist approach across all five English-speaking nations. Prior to IALS, basic skills education was run along national lines, meaning there was very little similarity between nations (Mendelovits, 2011; NRDC, 2011; Machin and Vignoles, 2006). After IALS, however, a common approach to adult basic skills was assumed, transforming literacy, numeracy and ESOL into content-based accredited courses with standardized curricula. This development allowed basic skills qualifications to be incorporated within the newly introduced national qualifications frameworks. These changes to basic skills education were part of a wider and arguably ideological restructuring in education which resulted in a single approach across the West, re-aligning the content and purpose of all education and training to better serve global capitalism in the twenty-first century (Milana and Nesbit, 2015; Green, 2002).

This restructuring of basic education played a crucial role in the functionalist orientation and development of health literacy because, unlike inter-active or critical health literacy, it claimed to be measurable (Haun et al., 2014; Nutbeam, 2008). Measurability, as we have outlined, is vitally important in providing positivist forms of evidence for outcomes-based healthcare systems and so would, in part, explain why FHL rather than IHL or CHL took off. Apart from the USA which tends to favour the use of diagnostic tools, e.g. the Rapid Estimate of Adult Health Literacy in Medicine (REALM), the Test Of Functional Health Literacy in Adults (TOFHLA) or the Newest Vital Sign (NVS), FHL's measurability largely rests upon the logic of accreditation; that is to say, where participation in accredited health-related learning (e.g. Skilled for Health) results in improved general literacy skills *and* improved knowledge about health as evidenced by *certification*.

But if health literacy means the ability to *act* on health information – not merely understand it – how do qualifications evidence action? This assumed linear relationship between knowing and doing is a recurring theme in health communication and one that needs further work to discover more precisely the nature of that relationship. Taking a critical realist stance, we suggest that unless information and knowledge are realized *through action* the evidence of health literacy will remain elusive. If people do engage in action, what then? What do we mean by an *act*? Does it mean a change in attitude or behaviour, and if it does mean either or both, how would these be measured as proof of being literate in health? Weintraub et al. (2004) believe one measure would be the increased ability of patients to 'participate fully in treatment decision-making processes' (Weintraub et al., 2004, cited in Corcoran, 2011: 75), but this kind of outcome would be very cumbersome to evidence using the positivist methods that currently dominate monitoring and evaluation frameworks in Western public health. Such instances of patient confidence and self-assertiveness would in any case be rare given the power dynamic that infuses the majority of patient–clinician relationships (Cuban, 2006). Self-confident, vocal and pro-active patients from the ranks of the disadvantaged are also an unlikely prospect for other reasons associated with educational exclusion in general and the unique journey of the adult learner in particular, to which we now turn.

Disadvantage, literacy and health

Health literacy – or the lack of it – is premised upon educational disadvantage which is recognized as a social determinant of health (Rowlands, 2012). This link has been established across North America and in Europe, but is nowhere so stark as in the UK (Dorling, 2015; Pickett and Wilkinson, 2009). Writing at the time when health literacy re-emerged as a 'new' concept in the 1990s, Sargant et al. (1997) reported a 'learning divide' between those adults who could easily access and afford post-compulsory education and those who could not. Although tackling educational disadvantage was high on the agenda of the New Labour government at the time the situation worsened and the inequalities gap is today wider and deeper than ever (Dorling, 2015; Pickett and Wilkinson, 2009). The pursuit of neoliberal policies has played a significant role in this, further disadvantaging those already disadvantaged, putting their modest aspirations beyond reach as increasing privatization of the sector demands a fee – even when subsidized.

Moreover, there are the participation costs to consider: travel, stationery, time etc., the associated costs of learning that the low-paid and unwaged can ill-afford. So while it is *possible* for the adult learner with low literacy skills to put a tentative foot on the first rung of the educational ladder, it is improbable. However, fees aren't the only challenge facing adult learners with low literacy: class; gender; age; educational experience; confidence and geography are bona fide reasons for not engaging in education (Sargant et al., 1997; Sargant and Aldridge, 2002). Then there is the issue of pedagogy, which has seen the virtual disappearance of andragogy in adult education and a return to traditional schooling methods which teach not through motivation, experience or indeed inspiration (Jarvis, 1987) but through incremental, bite-sized learning objectives that are evidenced using competency-based frameworks (Young, 2005). This is a frightful prospect for the 'non-learner' as they are often labelled, consigning mature students to a lengthy, disempowering process that, according to Young, makes them 'even less able to engage in more structured learning' (Young, 2005: 25).

This highlights two important issues for the FHL agenda of improving adult skills: firstly, it suggests that the target audience for FHL interventions will be reticent to engage voluntarily in *any* form of learning and secondly, that the performative processes of credentialism and marketization within post-compulsory education (accelerated by accreditation frameworks) will probably exclude the most disadvantaged from learning. Seen in this context, education can 'no longer be considered the vehicle for securing greater social equity' (Field, 2006: 101) which begs the question: is there any real point to improving basic literacies – including health literacy – through qualifications? Some may argue that the merit of FHL lies in offering second chance educational opportunities for those that missed out the first time around, or that gaining a recognized basic healthcare qualification will improve their career progression, but as O'Rourke highlights, this kind of offer in adult education 'only work[s] for people who are actively seeking access and opportunities' (O'Rourke, 1995, cited in Mayo and Thompson, 1995: 111).

The problem with FHL is its 'fuzzy' logic: it conflates literacy with knowledge, knowledge with action and action with good health which greatly over-simplifies the complexity of health communication and its relationship to action. While there is evidence to suggest links between multiple deprivation and poor health (Department of Health, 1980; Acheson, 1998; Marmot, 2006; WHO, 2007; Benzeval et al., 2014), the links between education, poor health and health literacy are less clear and it would be a mistake to simply link the two in a causal relationship, as FHL does. Part of the problem here is the nature of the evidence which is too disparate and unreliable to draw generalizable conclusions (Marshall, 2012). As Marshall points out, 'while conclusions [have been] made regarding health literacy levels in the population groups studied, there was often no indication of how these levels were determined, i.e. the established screening tools were rarely employed' (2012: 35). A big part of the problem relates to the multiple definitions of health literacy and the lack of conceptual clarity about the term, giving rise to epistemological as well as ontological problems in health literacy research (Rudd, 2015; Pleasant et al., 2011).

Despite these problems, educational achievement and health status continue to be linked because it is politic to do so. To do otherwise would mean shifting the blame from the individual onto more structural causes and with it, depositing the responsibility for righting the wrongs of inequality and injustice squarely upon the shoulders of political leaders. If the key determinants of health were given their due weight we might witness a completely different approach to health literacy: one that focuses not on proxy and imperfect indicators of disadvantage as in FHL, but a definition of health literacy in line with empowerment so that the 'causes of the causes' (WHO, 2007: 17) might be addressed. FHL cannot address the 'causes of the causes' that give rise to poor health literacy because it does not consider the 'key variables' at work between literacy and health outcomes (Rudd, 2015). With its singular focus on basic skills FHL offers a deficit model that targets and tests individuals in order to remedy what they apparently lack – and what they lack is good cognition. FHL's primary concerns are therefore to diagnose and improve the 'immediate barriers' that appear to be related to low-level cognition. This is a contestable notion. Consider for a moment some of the disabling effects old age, immaturity, developmental delay, trauma, impairment, illness and isolation might have on cognition. Even the context in which individual health literacy is measured (diagnostic tests and basic skills examinations) might well impair ability due to nerves or embarrassment. Moreover, while some of the examples cited might be permanent conditions – others are not. How does FHL account for the human condition if the agenda consistently fails to pay attention to the social nature of interaction and the context in which that interaction occurs?

FHL is inherently flawed as we have argued, but perhaps its biggest failing has been to treat the significant amount of data about the key determinants of health as mere artefact. Advancing individualist rhetoric and positivist instruments of measurement in the face of such a reality is unjust and does a disservice to those most in need. For this reason a more empowering, critical approach to health literacy is needed, one that at the very least, 'reminds us to consider individuals within multiple layers of the physical, social, and political systems over time' (Rudd, 2015: 7) and offers, 'a better hope for sustainable and equitable outcomes' (Baum, 2002).

Developing critical health literacy for health conscientization

It is clear from our discussion that FHL is problematic and why, for the reasons illustrated, it is not suited to making the level of impact where it is desired most. For health literacy to tangibly improve a radical alternative is required, one that is inclusive and which deals directly with the root causes of health inequalities – not just among the member states of the OECD – but across the industrializing and unindustrialized world. Alongside attempts to genuinely improve people's understanding of health and access to healthcare services throughout the lifecourse a critical, social and engaging form of health literacy needs to be developed; one that invites people to explore and act upon their health concerns. Critical health literacy (CHL) should therefore be a completely different kind of health literacy practice from what we have come to understand, a kind of practice that is supportive and participatory, making use of enactive forms of health communication where people can learn and become literate in health through experience. Thus, at the heart of CHL is the much maligned concept of empowerment (see Chapter 3), a powerful notion that, in the field of health literacy, has become lost in the wider debate (Sykes et al., 2013).

Critical health literacy has long been associated with empowerment (Sykes et al., 2013; Kickbusch, 2009, 2001) as this definition from the Worfld Health Organization illustrates:

Cognitive and social skills which determine the motivation and ability of individuals to gain access to, understand and use information in ways which promote and maintain good health. This means more than being able to read pamphlets and make appointments. By improving people's access to health information and their capacity to use it effectively, health literacy is critical to empowerment. (WHO, 2009)

Perhaps it is for this reason why CHL has struggled to get off the page and into practice, for empowerment – in its purest form – is a political act. Synonymous with Freire, empowerment is a form of collective education that has successfully addressed literacy issues through political awareness raising, enabling ordinary men and women to acquire a critical comprehension of their social reality (Freire, 1978: 24). Using dialogue as the method, people are encouraged within a group to critically explore the socio-cultural reality that shapes their lives and, rather more importantly, find solutions to transform that reality (Jarvis, 1987). Freire termed this process *conscientization* and it is this action-oriented collective process we need to adopt and take forward as the guiding principle in CHL – a form of 'health conscientization' if you will.

Implication for Practice 4

Western models of health often emphasize the role and responsibilities of the individual. What are the implications of this for professional praxis and how does this sit with an empowerment model of critical health literacy?

The role of health promoter would be key in the process of health conscientization, acting as a facilitator to gain a deeper understanding of the health concerns of those in the group. As with Freirean empowerment, concerns may well start off at the personal individual level, but they may also include concerns at the community or neighbourhood level, a regional or national level or touch on global health issues which affect the whole of humankind. Through critical dialogue the causes of these issues could be explored. This process generates socially constructed knowledge – a form of 'really useful knowledge' (Johnson, 1979) that communicates to the facilitator what health issues are important to the group. The original definition of 'really useful knowledge' is given in Chapter 3, but in terms of health communication for health promotion we can easily adapt this definition to provide a useful starting point for critical discussion. Really useful knowledge in this instance would be about the key factors that influence health and well-being, including a knowledge of why you get sick, and why through the force of social and economic circumstance you cannot expect to live a long and healthy life, but instead face the prospect of managing multiple long-term conditions with the likelihood that you could lose up to fifteen years of life.

Developing critical health literacy through experience

Besides Freirean dialogue, the health communicator might also consider using an experiential approach to develop CHL. Rudd's (2010) 'walking interview' is an excellent example of this, providing a structured learning experience which has potential benefit for both the healthcare provider and service user. The 'walking interview' is an exercise in which participants with any level of literacy explore the accessibility of a healthcare service or venue. Referring to a prescribed schedule, participants attempt to fulfil a range of tasks that test accessibility, for example asking for advice at the reception desk or trying to locate the public toilets. The responses are logged by one participant who acts as a scribe. If the process is undertaken using paper rather than electronic tools with voice recognition, it is recommended that the scribe have a good level of literacy. If working with people with very low literacy abilities this role might best be performed by the health promoter. If, however, the group has mixed level abilities then the practitioner may want to seize an opportunity to enhance the skills within the group by asking one of the group members to perform the role. In order to minimize the prospect of misinterpretation, the tasks are phrased in unambiguous language. The role of the scribe is to read out the tasks as set and log the answers faithfully against a range of preset options which allows for the data gathered to be compared against other datasets in a robust manner.

The process is as educative as it is illuminating, building participants' knowledge about healthcare services and treatments in a very practical way. What is more, there are potential benefits for the healthcare provider as findings from the exercise can be shared and used for service improvement or re-design. Participatory approaches such as this require the ability to structure an intervention well, and to consider the needs from both service users and providers to ensure that the intervention is fit for purpose and that it does not interfere with organizational business. Although originally designed by Rudd (2010) to test the accessibility of healthcare facilities for users with low literacy, minor modifications could expand the use of this model for application to a broader range of situations.

Developing critical health literacy through community development

As we have already highlighted in some detail, it is essential for effective health communication that practitioners develop a sound professional knowledge which is augmented by a practical, working knowledge about the nature of disadvantage in communities. Practitioners must also develop their practical expertise in the 'wicked competencies' and illustrate their commitment to empowering communities by demonstrating an ability to pursue and maintain respectful egalitarian relationships. Besides these considerable skills, we also suggest practitioners be effective networkers, organizers, lobbyists and excellent strategists who are capable of building high level, multi-disciplinary relationships to bring about a change in policies that directly affect the key determinants of health. Sykes et al. (2013) believe these skills uniquely define critical health literacy and are vital if practitioners are to communicate and interact in an empowering way. This is not new territory for radical practitioners in other disciplines, e.g. social work, adult education and community development; neither is it for the five English-speaking nations in focus here as each can reference their own rich and lengthy traditions. So in consideration of the recent calls for further research and wider discussion to examine how CHL may be developed in practice (Sykes et al., 2013), health promoters should consider the practices of those disciplines and build on what we know already works to develop a distinct form of *health conscientization* that would be locally inspired yet globally applicable.

However, if a radical community development approach were to be the direction of travel as so many health literacy commentators of late suggest it should be (Kickbusch, 2009; Nutbeam, 2008; WHO, 2009), the biggest obstacle facing CHL is not so much how to do it, but how to do it with the support of governments whose neoliberal policies actively contribute to, and widen health inequalities? Under the banner of austerity it is unlikely that a community development approach to CHL will be commissioned in the near future, especially considering the impact public service cuts have had upon the community development workforce. Community development has not fared well within public health departments and community development workers are often the first victims of funding cuts. The insistence on positivist forms of evidence would actively thwart a community development approach to CHL, perverting it instead to another form of functional health literacy which would increase the incidence of short-term project work aimed at behaviour change, reducing the capacity for working upstream in a holistic way for the long term.

That said, this need not hinder or deter any *practical* efforts to bring CHL about for it is through our daily actions that we breathe life into such commitments. How else can health practitioners change the narrow confines of their current working environment to effect real, long lasting transformations at an individual, community and societal level? Only by working strategically to raise awareness and foster agency in ordinary communities will health promoters genuinely contribute to a social movement in health promotion and make good on the promise of tackling health inequalities at source in a truly empowering way. Archer's (1995) theory of human agency is insightful here and is worthy of consideration because, without reducing the complexity of the issues, she offers a critical realist perspective into how agency is first formed, under what conditions it flourishes and how it may be directed and used to effect structural change. Archer's theory succeeds in telling the story of how people make history, but more importantly how they might go about fashioning a different future. There is a key part for health promoters to play here because by virtue of their professional role they are suitably positioned within organizations to advance particular agendas. Archer's theory of human agency sits perfectly with the educational and psycho-social theories presented in this book and, if taken up, would enable practitioners to nurture a critical and transformative form of health literacy to empower.

Summary of key points

This chapter has provided a critical historical overview of health literacy, highlighting key debates within the literature that inform its continuous evolution. Specifically it has:

- given a brief overview of the competing and divergent definitions of health literacy
- examined the origins of functionalism within functional health literacy

- presented a generic critique of FHL tools
- considered the suitedness of FHL to radical health promotion praxis
- explored how key concepts and theories in health promotion can support the development of critical health literacy

> **Reflection 1** – As a professional or lay person, are you able to identify practices in healthcare provision that have been informed by the concept of health literacy? Can you identify what definition of health literacy was in operation? How effective were the health messages?

> **Reflection 2** – As we have established within the chapter, readability is a particularly popular method used in functional health literacy that Hoffman and McKenna (2006) could be expanded to educate the public by stealth. How would you improve readability?

> **Reflection 3** – How might critical health literacy look in practice? What kinds of multi-disciplinary relationships might you need to foster if working on an agenda that aims to tackle the wider determinants of health? What kinds of networks outside your professional discipline exist to support the development of critical health literacy?

> **Reflection 4** – The majority of activity in health literacy is currently located in the West. Do you think it is a transferable concept to other parts of the world? If so, what particular form of health literacy do you think would be most beneficial and how?

Further reading

Kickbusch, I. (2009) Health literacy: engaging in a political debate. *International Journal of Public Health*, 131–2.
In this article Kickbusch argues for a new form of health citizenship in which citizens take personal responsibility for health and become involved in social and political processes that address the root causes of health inequalities, as well as inequalities in access to care.
Tones, K. (2002) Health literacy: new wine in old bottles? *Health Education Research*, 17 (3), 287–90.
In this article Tones explores the meaning of health literacy proper, and challenges the appropriateness of using the term to redefine territory that has already been mapped by existing conceptualizations of individual and community empowerment.

Rudd, R. (2010) The Health Literacy Environment Activity Packet: *First Impressions and a Walking Interview*.

This packet focuses on four activities designed to help staff members consider the health literacy environment of their workplace. First impressions focus on the phone, the web and the walk to the facility. The walking interview is a navigation exercise.

Part III

Issues and Challenges

8
Challenges in Health Communication and Behaviour Change

Key aims

- To critically consider the concept of health behaviour as social practice
- To examine how we might communicate health to different people within different contexts taking into account the process and structural barriers which may arise when communicating health messages
- To critically consider how health inequality might be addressed and acknowledge the social inequity that people face
- To acknowledge and examine some of the ethical challenges faced in health communication
- To critically consider Nudge Theory and Choice Architecture

Introduction

This chapter takes a more critical approach to the concept of behaviour change and the issues and challenges that health promoters face in communicating health messages to a diverse population. It will outline the key challenges that exist adopting a more analytical approach to the notion of behaviour. It draws on examples from the wider literature to consider what challenges are faced and how these might be overcome to promote better health outcomes. It therefore considers alternative ways of thinking about behaviour and behaviour change discussing ideas about 'health behaviours' in contrast with notions of 'social practices'. It examines communication issues relating to factors such as culture, gender and age focusing on issues arising from communicating with different groups of people in different contexts. The chapter considers process and structural barriers communicating health messages and the more recent ideas of Nudge Theory and Choice Architecture. Finally it includes an appraisal of ethical issues in health communication such as those associated with dilemmas in persuasive and coercive communication, and the challenges that such methods pose to concerns within empowerment.

Health behaviour as social practice – implications for health communication

Individual health behaviour is an aspect of health under frequent and recurring examination particularly in the current neoliberal political climate in the UK and other similar contexts. We observe that this is a pattern which is being replicated in other countries across the globe. This is reflected in health policy and health strategies increasingly using social marketing approaches to public health which ultimately focus on behavioural change at an individual level (French et al., 2010) as discussed in more detail in Chapter 6.

The argument that we should perhaps rethink the whole concept of 'health behaviour/s' was introduced in Chapter 4. As highlighted, there are some critics of this term who have proposed that we shift focus away from individual health behaviour and the reliance on social cognition models to understand it (Mielewczyk and Willig, 2007; Robertson and Williams, 2010). There is increasing recognition that human behaviours and interactions are extremely complex. As stated, Mielewczyk and Willig (2007) argue that 'health behaviours' do not exist. They acknowledge the term 'health-related behaviours' – however, their emphasis is on social context and the meaning that certain types of behaviours may have dependent on the context in which they take place. Given this emphasis, they suggest that the term 'social practice/s' should be used instead so that 'health behaviour' is reconceptualized and examined in relation to the wider social practices within which it takes place. This, Mielewczyk and Willig (2007) argue, would give greater emphasis to the meaning and functions which different practices serve the people who engage in them. There is, therefore, a need for a more critical perspective and greater recognition of the importance of lay perspectives. Importantly, challenging existing ideas about health behaviour enables us to raise questions about who is privileged and/or marginalized (and how) by the constructions which dominate our collective understanding of such things. We wrote in Chapter 1 about the need to trouble received wisdom. Challenging dominant constructions and discourse is a necessary way of achieving this. This chapter (and the following one) offer up a number of ways in which we do this.

We can turn again to critical psychology for a deeper appreciation of this perspective. Here we find the argument that the reason why individual health behaviour is so hard to predict is because there is no such thing; it is a 'fabrication' or 'made-up' phenomenon (Stainton-Rogers, 2011). Stainton-Rogers takes condom-use as an example to illustrate the problems in mainstream or traditional approaches to understanding and predicting health behaviours. She argues that condom-use research neglects to take account of the complexities of, for example, negotiation, expectations and relationships. If we apply a similar approach to alcohol-use we can appreciate that drinking alcohol will have different meanings for different people in different contexts at different times. It is difficult to draw comparisons between the motivations of, for example, a person who has the occasional glass of sparkling wine in a celebratory social situation and someone who sets out to achieve 'determined drunkenness', for whatever reason (Measham and Brain, 2005). This is referred to as situated social practice. How we communicate health messages about alcohol would be affected by the differences in these cases.

In 2014 a special issue of the international journal *Sociology of Health and Illness* was called 'From Health Behaviours to Health Practices: Critical Perspectives'. In it there were a number of excellent peer-reviewed sociological papers which explained this perspective. The papers contain a number of critiques of traditional understandings of health behaviour which mirror the critique presented in the themes throughout this book including deconstructing the notion of the rational actor, resisting determinism and recognition that health is created beyond the individual level within and through our wider environments and the structures of society. There is a challenge to the assumption that health behaviour is 'discrete, stable, homogenous and measurable' (Cohn, 2014: 157). There is a challenge to the neoliberal assumption that better health is achievable primarily through better self-management and informed choice (Horrocks and Johnson, 2014). There is debate about agency and structure and a consideration of these in the light of the practice of health promotion and public health (Veenstra and Burnett, 2014). There is a call for change in terms of focusing not only on a contextualized approach to understanding health practices but also on focusing on health unequities in a range of environmental conditions rather than health inequalities in outcomes (Frohlich and Abel, 2014). Notably Frohlich and Abel (2014) draw on social geography's concept of environmental injustice which 'underscores the moral nature of the spatial distribution of opportunities' (p. 199). Baum and Fisher (2014) point to the lack of consideration of social determinants of health in health policy and the lack of recognition that certain health behaviours are more common in different social strata. Importantly they highlight several ways in which a focus on individual behaviour is inappropriate for tackling social inequities. Ong et al. (2014) point to the fact that social context remains under-theorized and under-explored. Crucially Nettleton and Green (2014) argue that 'the sociology of public health needs to focus less on health behaviour and more on social practice' (p. 239). In the context of substance- and alcohol-use in pregnancy Benoit et al. (2014) contend that such practice is shaped by socio-cultural factors, notably that such behaviour is unacceptable. 'This framing of problematic substance use is accomplished via gendered responsibilization of women as foetal incubators and primary care givers of infants' (p. 252). A further paper in this collection is based on research carried out in Cameroon. In it van de Sijpt (2014) discussed the contextualization of reproductive behaviours and challenges neoliberal assumptions of choice, autonomy and control around fertility outcomes arguing that 'individual fertility intentions are often not the result of rational calculation and reproductive happenings do not exist in a social vacuum' (p. 278).

Importantly, this collection of arguments points to the significant limitations that traditional, or mainstream, understandings have for improving health outcomes and influencing policy as well as addressing the social determinants of health. Notably the empiri-cal papers within this special edition draw on qualitative research privileging the lay perspective which is crucial for developing such understanding. Framing health behaviours as 'health practices', it is argued, opens up greater opportunities for understanding and theorizing (Cohn, 2014). Taking such an approach also enables those working in health communication to challenge individualistic victim-blaming ideologies and the 'deviance' discourse that coheres around certain types of health behaviours framed as 'bad', 'undesir-able' and 'problematic'.

Communicating health to different groups in different contexts

Beginning with revelations of a landmark document, the Black Report (DHSS, 1980), reducing health inequalities has become a key issue in UK healthcare in the last thirty years. The report, at the time, received limited recognition and implementation due to a change in government from a left-wing one that commissioned it to a right-wing one that was hostile to the report's political and social premise. In the intervening decades the policy process has shifted from neoliberal (Thatcher) to managerial (Major) to modernizing (early New Labour) to user-focused (later New Labour) back to neoliberal (Coalition and then Cameron). One constant throughout this time has been the premise that delivery has been difficult because of so-called 'hard-to-reach' population groups. For example, one of the key messages in the 2002 UK Department of Health document in 'Addressing inequality – reaching the hard to reach groups' (DH, 2002) is about using different strategies to target health promotion messages and services at different 'hard-to-reach' populations. Although it is agreed that actions to address health inequalities need a broad-based approach, services are often targeted at marginalized, vulnerable, disadvantaged and deprived groups. By 2008, the health of the most disadvantaged groups in society had not improved as fast as the better off. The health gap had actually widened. This was problematic as seen in the documents 'Health Inequalities: progress and next steps' (DH, 2008) and Fair Society, Healthy Lives, The Marmot Review (Marmot, 2010). People at the higher socio-economic rungs of the ladder were the ones benefitting from the strategies. Reducing health inequalities is a matter of fairness and social justice. The Marmot Review suggests that 'focusing solely on the most disadvantaged will not reduce health inequalities sufficiently. To reduce the steepness of the social gradient in health, actions must be universal, but with a scale and intensity that is proportionate to the level of disadvantage. We call this proportionate universalism' (Marmot, 2010: 9).

As health promoters, we work with very diverse populations; differences in age, gender, ethnicity, religion, disability and sexuality. All individuals have specific needs and values. There is a consensus in all of these strategies and reports that healthcare provision needs to be culturally sensitive and appropriate, meeting the needs of the public. Communicating health messages effectively depends on the design of communication strategies in meeting the needs of the population group. In the UK since 2007, local authorities have had a statutory requirement to produce a Joint Strategic Needs Assessment annually and this is central to commissioning services for its population (DH, 2007). Although there are guidelines on the Health Needs Assessment process, the decision about whose need is a priority is not always clear. While making our assessment of needs, how can we ensure services are 'proportionately universal'? More importantly, how do we design health promotion activities accessible to all, but with a scale and intensity to the level of disadvantage, as recommended by the Marmot Review (Marmot, 2010)?

It is inevitable that some sections of the population will be 'targeted'. They may be people who are seen as somehow different in terms of stigma and social exclusion in a healthcare context. In the context of health promotion and communicating health messages, they may be the sections of the population with normative needs as described by Bradshaw (1972) and who are difficult to reach by health promoters. They may consider themselves healthy and see no reason to contact health services; for example, healthy young people, healthy working adults, travellers, black and minority ethnic communities. In this sense, they are hard to reach from the health promotion service point of view; the difficulties lie with the health promoter, not with the population themselves.

The term 'hard-to-reach' has become a commonly used term to address specific groups of the population who are hard to reach by service providers. Health and Safety Executive (HSE, 2004: 8) defined 'hard-to-reach' as people who are *inaccessible to most traditional and conventional methods for any reason'*. Although there is a lack of consensus in the meaning of the term, there is also a sense of negativity in reaching certain groups of people (Flanagan and Hancock, 2010). Flanagan and Hancock (2010) studied the notion of 'hard-to-reach' from the Voluntary and Community sector's point of view and the barriers and facilitators in service accessibility. It is suggested that 'hard-to-reach' groups are people who are, in some ways, more needy; more marginalized; more likely to have experienced poverty, whether that be economic poverty or poverty of opportunity, non-service users, the non-engaged, and people who have 'fallen through the net'. Again, the term 'hard-to-reach' is a service-centred point of view rather than coming from communities themselves. The respondents in Flanagan and Hancock's (2010) study did recognize that the barriers for non-engagement could have been put up by the service provider and the system rather than the public (e.g. previous negative experiences, service location and time, lack of information, lack of choices). The term may infer blame and lead to prejudice and discrimination (Corcoran, 2013). Certain groups can be stigmatized or even oppressed in the way that they are included or excluded, or left out by simply being overlooked as a result of targeted services. The term 'hard-to-reach' can imply that this is the major problem that the group or community face.

In a study on service commissioning in London by Mauger et al. (2010), strategic commissioners said they wanted to involve 'hard-to-reach groups' in commissioning. However, the researchers found that commissioners didn't really talk directly to many user groups. Actually, for commissioners, everyone was hard to reach! The risk is that if services do seek out to 'hard-to-reach' groups, this can be a negative rather than positive step. In a study about advocacy for Black Mental Health service users (Rai-Atkins, 2002), it was clear (a) that mainstream services had real difficulties in even knowing about minority communities in their own areas, (b) that the services being made available were usually very unsuitable for minority communities and (c) being hard to reach often proved to be a bonus for some communities – it meant that they were given money to provide their own (much more appropriate) support. This is a sombre finding replicated in more recent studies (Beresford et al., 2010; Beresford et al., 2016 forthcoming) and opens up a complex discussion about mainstreaming versus community-centred support. A project on Power Analysis (Hunjan and Keophilavong, 2010; Hunjan and Pettit, 2011) suggested that groups deemed to be excluded and/or without power should analyse their own power and the power around them. Services seeing groups as 'hard-to-reach' might indicate closed or manipulated spaces of which user groups should be wary and the groups may better focus on the power they already have and create their own claimed spaces. In one sense, services using the term 'hard-to-reach' can indicate a problem with (and for) the services. The type of change required should therefore be about changing attitudes and culture within services (Forrest et al., 2013).

In the light of this, health communication efforts need to be culturally tailored based on an understanding of a particular group's beliefs and values, traditions, lifestyle and philosophies. For example, culture can be an important audience-segmentation variable in health communication design (Kreuter and McClure, 2004). In addition, language and gender can also be process barriers as can challenges raised by people with a physical impairment or mental health issues. In the same way, difficulties may arise because of structural and environmental barriers. For example, the way health organizations work, how services are provided, how policies are implemented as well as the awareness of societal factors such as social class, access to education and literacy levels. Health inequalities are often driven by social inequities. Addressing all of this, a progressive health communication strategy needs to be authentic and appropriate to the communities or groups concerned. Simplistic labels and stereotypes are not enough. To understand the complexity of health inequality and population health, Bauer (2014) argued that the concept of intersectionality has much to offer in the identification of health inequality and the development of intervention strategies. According to Bowleg (2012), individuals (at the micro level) have multiple intersecting social identities such as race, gender, disability, socio-economic status, which also intersect with the multiple levels of social inequalities such as sexism and racism at the macro structural level resulting in a complex web of social inequality. Intersectionality therefore provides an interpretive and analytical framework for understanding and addressing disparities and social inequalities in health.

To improve the accessibility of services, the lack of funding and issues in partnership-working such as the relationship between statutory and voluntary sectors also feature strongly in Flanagan and Hancock's (2010) study. This study emphasized the importance of involving the public's *choices* and *voices*. The study indicated that the four areas which need attention are the attitudes of staff; service flexibility; working in partnership with other organizations; and empowering and involving service users. In a review by Coles et al. (2012) on community-based health and health promotion for homeless people, a tailored approach to the design of interventions was suggested. The psychosocial needs and life circumstances of the population group should therefore be incorporated into the development of the intervention. This review dovetails with Flanagan and Hancock's

(2010) in that the case for the *active* involvement and participation of the beneficiaries of any intervention is clear. In order for services (or health communication efforts) to be accessible and effective the intended beneficiaries must be meaningfully involved at every stage of the process.

The challenge remains in addressing health inequalities and social inequity in neoliberal Western societies where the narrative is presented as simply being about personal freedom and individual control. Is a 'behaviour change' approach necessary, sufficient, or should it even be a priority to promote health through health communication if the fundamental causes of inequity are not individual but are political, global, structural and essentially about the unequal distribution of power and resources?

Implication for Practice 2

It is crucial to consider what issues may arise when we focus on a particular group or community. We need to think about how certain groups may be stigmatized or even oppressed, or how other groups may be left out by simply being overlooked as a result of this focusing.

Implication for Practice 3

It is important to consider how models of behaviour might underpin health communication practice. Consider whether your practice needs to change in order to take into account the structural barriers that people may encounter.

Ethics and health communication

The core purpose of health promotion is to enable *communities* to take control of their own health (WHO, 1986) and we believe the best way to achieve this is to nurture agency through practices that are ethical and empowering (see Chapter 3). However, in the current context of professional practice there are some challenging implications associated with this, especially where the health agenda is driven by central state policy rather than local communities; is informed by the bioethics of a clinical model rather than the broader macro-ethical framework of the social model (Sindall, 2002), and where health promotion interventions are designed for efficacy and value for money and evaluated against distorted notions of public accountability that use positivist methods such as outcomes-based frameworks (see Chapter 9).

This discourse, which dominates public health in the West, favours models of behaviour change in health improvement and as such is wholly irreconcilable with empowerment (Tengland, 2012). This is because models of behaviour change target the individual rather than the collective and because they privilege professional 'expert' knowledge, thereby increasing professional autonomy and 'top-down' forms of health communication at the expense of the laity's knowledge, experience and engagement. Crucially, theories of behaviour change disregard the socio-economic and political factors that empowering approaches to improving health consider fundamental, making them resonate with the individualist social ontology of neoliberalism that blames the victim for their poor 'lifestyle choices' (Yeo, 1993).

In this setting, the radical practitioner finds themselves in an ethical quandary: how are they to realize the principles and values that guide emancipatory health promotion praxis when they are stranded within professional structures that thwart just that? However, according to the literature (Williamson, 2014; Tannahill, 2008; Sindall, 2002; Yeo, 1993; Last, 1987) the real problem is not the professional structures in which the work takes place, but the professional culture of health promotion – and more specifically the lack of a code of ethics to distinguish its unique purpose and methods from medical and other allied health professionals: a code of communitarian ethics that 'moves beyond the principles derived from bioethics, to incorporate theories from social and political philosophy' (Sindall, 2002).

Given the political climate (see Chapter 9), it is questionable whether a code of ethics would improve this situation; after all, other professions that already ascribe to such a code have shown it to be of little use against the ideological restructuring of public services by the state. As Crowther (1995) highlights using examples from higher education, independent organizations that attempted to resist realigning their practices to government policy in the 1990s risked having their funds withdrawn or their professional licence revoked. What this example also illustrates is just how little opportunity there is to meaningfully subvert the neoliberal agenda, leaving radical practitioners everywhere with a choice of either adapting their ethical commitments to better suit trends in policy, or continuing with a purist radical agenda *beyond* professional structures. Indeed, one might conclude from this that the real problem lies with the concept of professionalism itself, which ultimately promotes a set of values and practices that is at odds with emancipatory praxis, rigorously controlling and excluding – as it is designed to do – access to specialist knowledge, prestige and power.

Yet, despite the dangers and difficulties for the radical practitioner (Green et al., 2015) there is always the possibility to do transformational work – even in environments that are marked by limitation and constraint, and the starting point for this is *dialogue*. Surely, the very restrictions on emancipatory praxis provide the important and authentic subject matter to initiate and enter into dialogue with lay people and professionals alike? This would raise awareness in a classical Freirean sense to inform a critical mass which, in turn, might trigger a powerful form of agency that Archer calls 'corporate power' (2000). Used strategically, corporate power has transformative powers at an organizational level and it may just well be the way forward for practitioners who do not want to have to choose between their principles or profession. That said, to acquire corporate power demands much of the radical practitioner, and the health promotion professional of the future must be both sufficiently knowledgeable and skilled to deploy the same range of sophisticated skills used in practice among key influencers in the political domain to defend and promote democratic, emancipatory praxis.

Persuasion, coercion and use of fear and emotive appeals

The methods used in health communication are many and varied, as illustrated by the examples in this book. Fear tactics are often used in efforts to promote health. Fear is explicitly used in health communication but it is also evident in more implicit ways. For example, the representation of the drunken woman as 'vulnerable' is a dominant contemporary discourse (Jackson and Tinkler, 2007). Highlighting women's vulnerability may produce a fear response which can serve as a powerful way of controlling behaviour (Sanders, 2006). Yet, this is inherently problematic. Not only does it play into gendered stereotypes, it also leads to victim-blaming.

Assumptions that behaviour change will occur as a consequence of receiving information about the detrimental effect of certain practices are ill-grounded; there is little in the way of evidence to support such assumptions. In addition, there has often been a deterministic, individualistic focus on 'bad' behaviours and unhealthy practices such as smoking for example (McKie et al., 2003). However, persuasive measures do not appear to be very effective, nor do those that are premised on fear or trying to change behaviour through provoking anxiety (Breakwell, 2007). As argued by Mielewczyk and Willig (2007) there needs to be a move away from trying to persuade or coerce people into changing certain targeted behaviours, to designing interventions which seek to explore the meanings which underpin different practices. In addition, interventions which are designed to explore the purpose that certain risky practices serve, and perhaps provide alternative strategies, might prove to be more effective. Public health and health promotion policy and practice should, ideally, aim to take into account the ways in which health practices are understood and the meanings which they have. For example, Robertson's (2006) study exploring men's concepts of risk and health showed that 'risky' lifestyle practices are socially integrated and take place within the context of everyday life.

We often use emotive appeals in health communication. Seldom is this more apparent than the issue of breastfeeding which is of global relevance. National policy derives from the recommendations of the World Health Organization which advocates exclusive breastfeeding for the first six months of life. Women are exhorted to exercise informed choice which is assumed to be available to them as a result of being educated about a range of issues concerned with child-bearing and child-rearing. The issue of coercion is relevant here. Contemporary constructions of motherhood position select particular choices as the 'right' choices (Phipps, 2014). Breastfeeding is just one example where this occurs – it is promoted as better than formula feed. The means by which this is done are varied, however, and maternal feelings are often manipulated in the process – 'if you want what's best for your infant you will choose to breastfeed'. The outcomes for women who don't are judgement, blame and shame. In fact, some health communication campaigns actually use shame and blame to promote breastfeeding. Phipps (2014) cites the example of the UK charity Save the Children which, in 2013, actually recommended putting cigarette-style warnings on packages of formula feed. The focus at the individual level of choice ignores structural factors which may come into play such as maternal benefits and the lack of opportunity to breastfeed in the workplace, for example. Those who possess greater capital (for example, social and economic) are often better placed to exercise choice and have relative access to privilege. Health communication efforts often play on people's insecurities and fears (Fischer and Lotz, 2014). Such efforts should be questioned from an ethical standpoint.

Personal anxieties are played upon in health communication efforts – fear of ill-health, fear of injury, or even, for example, fear of 'getting fat' and the associated social stigmatization that this brings with it. Health promotion campaigns often use fear to motivate behaviour change (Bradley, 2011). Questions can, and should, be raised as to the extent to which it is acceptable to use such methods and whether it is appropriate. There is inconclusive evidence as to whether fear-based approaches are more effective in promoting behaviour change as compared with, for example, approaches using humour or positive messages. People are more likely to disengage with and ignore messages when their anxiety is raised too high. It is also ethically questionable to cause stress and distress as a means to an end. As pointed out by Maguire (2006) fear is often used paternalistically to change behaviour. Maguire refers to the use of fear as a 'technology of governance', an argument that nicely dovetails with our discussion of governance in the following chapter – Chapter 9. The manipulation of emotions in health communication is clearly the result of coercive power. People differ in their ability to contest and resist such power. This is often related to structural factors in society such as relative disadvantage and inequality.

Implication for Practice 4

As practitioners in health communication it is important to be aware of the ethical implications of what we do. At times the ends may justify the means; however, maintaining a reflective approach to practice is crucial in order to be aware of, and address, any ethical concerns.

Nudge Theory and Choice Architecture

In this section we set out to consider Nudge Theory and the concept of Choice Architecture. To begin with it is necessary to give a very brief overview of what these are and how they are inextricably linked. Thaler and Sunstein (2008) first put forward the notion of 'nudge' in their book *Nudge: Improving Decisions about Health, Wealth and Happiness*. They define it as 'any aspect of the choice architecture that alters people's behaviour in a predictable way without forbidding any options or significantly changing their economic intentions'. Specifically they state that, 'to count as a mere nudge, the intervention must be easy and cheap to avoid. Nudges are not mandates. Putting fruit at eye level counts as a nudge. Banning junk food does not' (p. 6). More succinctly, Oliver (2013: 1) states that 'nudge is a non-regulatory approach that attempts to motivate individual behaviour change through subtle alterations in the choice environments that people face'. Choice architecture is therefore about altering circumstances or environments to promote healthier choices while not restricting personal freedom. Those that do so are referred to as 'choice architects'.

We can differentiate between different types of nudges as defined by the Local Government Association (2013):

- Provision of information – for example, calorie counts on menus
- Changes to environment – for example, designing buildings with fewer lifts
- Changes to default – making salad the default option instead of chips (french fries)
- Use of norms – providing information about what others are doing.

Nudge theory and choice architecture are rooted in behavioural economics which is concerned with understanding how people behave. Perhaps unsurprisingly, it has gained significant ground in 'Western' countries in recent years. Specialized units have been set up in the UK, the USA and Australia in order to direct policy and practice which aims to influence behaviour at individual, group and community levels. The assumption underpinning nudge theory is that motivation and behaviour can be influenced via a number of indirect mechanisms that can work as well as direct ones such as removing choice and telling people what to do. Although nudge theory and choice architecture have generally been accepted relatively unquestioningly, from a critical perspective the concepts raise a number of issues that are worth exploring. Using 'unconscious' processes to mould behaviour undermines empowerment approaches. Empowerment is, of course, a central plank of health promotion. There is an ethical concern here also.

Nudges often operate on a subconscious or unconscious level. This has been described as a form of covert coercion (Local Government Association, 2013; Oliver, 2013) and is unacceptable to some. This contrasts with the supposed *voluntary* nature of the nudge concept. Oliver (2013) gives the following example of this apparent contradiction in terms – 'if people are meant to face the changes in the choice architecture unconsciously – e.g. unconsciously face fruit rather than cheesecake at eye level as they are about to pay for their lunch in their local canteen – how can they make the conscious decision of non-participation?'. In theory the concept of nudge or choice architecture privileges the neoliberal notion of free will and the exercise of choice by not removing or restricting it. However, the nudge takes away conscious choice. Oliver (2013) argues that 'if the nudge is made explicit it might be actively resisted! A dilemma thus ensues: it may be that the only way that a nudge will work is via a level of covertness that many might deem unacceptable from a democratic government' (p. 3).

The politics of nudge is also open to question. Nudge is being used to drive forward the domestic policy agendas around public health led by the respective governments in both the USA and the UK. Interestingly, these two agendas reflect similar policy despite the apparent lack of parity in political perspectives between the two governments. Perhaps this is a case of jumping on the band wagon. Boyce et al. (2008) specifically criticizes nudge as being a short-term, politically motivated initiative which is unsupported by substantive evidence. Notably, nudge theory does not take into account the wider determinants of health but also psychological determinants of health. In keeping with one of the central critiques presented within this book Frerichs (2011) criticizes policy based on nudge for its focus on the behavioural symptoms that arise from economic and social determinants. Ménard (2010) adds to this by pointing out the individualistic focus and the lack of attention to issues of social justice.

Given the political interest in nudge in driving forward policy agendas it is clear to see that the choice architecture is being used to promote behaviours which are desired by the state at the expense of individual freedom and autonomy (Schnellenbach, 2012). Choice architectures (or those that advise them) are positioned as the 'experts' within this model. These 'experts' are the people who possess the knowledge about what behaviour is 'correct'. This raises questions as to the extent to which state or government intervention at the individual behaviour level is acceptable, particularly when it comes to health (Ménard, 2010). Nudges therefore 'subject us to the control of others because of the mechanisms through which they operate' (Saghai, 2013: 487).

It is assumed that behaviour can be changed through 'nudges'. The question, from an ethical point of view, is whether it *should* be (Fischer and Lotz, 2014). Wilkinson (2013) argues that 'nudges can manipulate, even if the aim is to benefit the victim or society and even though, by definition, they come with the formal freedom to opt out' (p. 354) particularly if those who are targeted by the nudge are not fully cognizant or consenting of it. Fischer and Lotz (2014) critique the notion of 'soft paternalism' (or libertarian paternalism) inherent in nudge theory. Notably, the idea of libertarian paternalism can be seen as a contradiction in terms (Cross et al., 2013).

Fischer and Lotz (2014) also question nudge from an ethical standpoint. They argue that the term nudge is 'conceptually vague and possibly not coherent' (p. 2) and criticize the broad-brush approach to understanding human behaviour which, they argue, is far more complex than nudge allows for. In addition, they point to the problems inherent in the lack of mutual appreciation of 'heavily contested normative terms' such as 'freedom' and 'wellbeing' (p. 2) which, they argue, adds to the lack of clarity and understanding. We would suggest that 'autonomy' should be added to these terms.

Fischer and Lotz (2014) contend that criticisms of nudges are two-fold. Firstly, linked to utilitarianism, nudge reduces an individual's capacity for control over action. Secondly, linked to Kantian ethics, individual autonomy is 'interfered with' (p. 4). Ménard (2010) poses the questions as to whether it is 'possible to interfere with individual decision-making while preserving freedom of choice' (p. 229). Both criticisms link back to fundamental principles of health promotion outlined in this book such as empowerment and participation. Clearly such principles are undermined when using choice architecture approaches in health communication and behaviour change. The question then becomes, does the end justify the means?

A commentary in the UK newspaper the *Guardian* pointed to the critique that nudges can infantilize individuals by taking away their moral maturity (Chalabi, 2013). This position is borne out through the terminology used in a document produced by the Local Government Association which refers to other techniques for changing behaviour (alongside 'nudging') – 'techniques like direct incentives, such as vouchers in return for healthy behaviour, are being labelled hugs, while the tougher measures that restrict choice, like restricting takeaways from schools, are shoves. Bans, such as the restriction on smoking in public places, are simply known as smacks' (Local Government Association, 2013).

Some critics, such as Goodwin (2012), simply argue that we should reject the use of 'nudge'. Goodwin (2012) contends that nudge is contrary to notions of empowerment, freedom and fairness and that it fails to tackle wider issues. Bonell et al. (2011) argue that the right-wing UK government has misrepresented the nudge concept in an attempt to 'obscure the (government's) failure to propose realistic actions to address the upstream socio-economic and environmental determinants of health' (p. 2158). Instead, they argue, nudge focuses downstream on choices that are made at an individual level. Nudge's inability to address social determinants of health such as poverty has been highlighted (Allmark and Tod, 2013). In fact, a key critique of nudge and choice architecture is the lack of consideration of the socio-economic determinants of behaviour (Bonell et al., 2011). Allmark and Tod (2013), however, point to the potential for nudges to influence behaviour through environmental modifications with regard to excess winter deaths (an issue that reflects wider social determinants of health) alongside a range of other measures. In order to achieve this, 'a careful approach to nudges, adhering strictly to the level of transparency required in a democratic society, is needed to ensure that the outcomes pursued through nudges truly represent a societal consensus, and that nudges are not simply introduced as a technocratic short cut' (Fischer and Lotz, 2014: 14).

There is a lack of research and evidence at a population level on behaviour change interventions (Science and Technology Select Committee, 2011) particularly with regard to long-term effects. There is also a lack of a secure evidence base on nudge and choice architecture although there appears to be a general consensus that nudging works. Nudging may not be as effective as regulatory or legislative measures in shaping certain types of behaviour and this, in itself, is of concern if, for example, that behaviour causes harm to others. Nudge needs to be combined with other measures including regulatory ones. There appears to be general consensus that nudging is only part of the solution and not likely to be successful on its own. Finally, Oliver (2013) critiques nudge for being 'somewhat theoretically empty and, in practice, too often gimmicky'. Oliver proposes a new approach – *budge* not nudge. Budge is defined as 'behavioural economic-informed regulation designed to budge the private sector away from socially harmful acts' (Oliver, 2013) and seeks to determine better understandings of where and how to regulate in order for people to avoid harming themselves (or others).

Summary of key points

This chapter has discussed a number of key challenges in health communication. Specifically it has:

- critically considered the concept of health behaviour as social practice
- examined how we might communicate health to different people

within different contexts taking into account the process and structural barriers which may arise when communicating health messages

- critically considered how health inequality might be addressed and acknowledged the social inequity that people face
- examined some of the ethical challenges faced in health communication
- critically considered Nudge Theory and Choice Architecture

Reflection 1 – How would shifting understandings of 'health behaviours' to 'social practices' enable greater understanding of different public health issues? Choose one public health issue that interests you and consider what new emphases there would be. How would this difference in approach impact on health communication efforts in that area? At what level would action be potentially most effective?

Reflection 2 – Reflect on any so-called 'hard-to-reach' communities you have worked with in practice. Consider why these communities are labelled 'hard-to-reach'. How are they 'hard-to-reach' and why are they perceived to be that way? What process and structural barriers have you come across in relation to them? How could these be overcome?

Reflection 3 – All health communication efforts will involve ethical considerations of one sort or another. Select a specific health communication or health promotion intervention. What do you see as the key ethical concerns within it? From an ethical perspective consider the intended beneficiaries (and those who will not benefit), the methods used (are they acceptable and appropriate?) and the potential outcomes.

Reflection 4 – How might the concepts of nudge and choice architecture be applied to the area in which you work? What are the limitations of using this type of approach? What other things could be done to augment or improve effectiveness (think about this at structural levels if possible)?

Further reading

Corcoran, N. (2013) *Communicating Health: Strategies for Health Promotion.* 2nd edn. London: Sage.
This book presents a range of communication skills pertinent to promoting health. It contains a useful content highly relevant to some of the dis-

cussion in this chapter, specifically Chapter 3 – 'Reaching Unreachable Groups and Crossing Cultural Barriers'.

Marmot, M. (2010) *Fair Society Healthy Lives: The Marmot Review*. The Marmot Review. Strategy review of Health Inequality post 2010.

The Marmot Review outlines effective evidence-based strategies for addressing health inequalities. Focusing on the social determinants of health it has global relevance and presents a range of actions at policy level which have the potential to make a real difference to health outcomes.

Special issue of *Sociology of Health and Illness: From Health Behaviours to Health Practices: Critical Perspectives*. February 2014. Volume 36, Issue 2.

This special issue focuses specifically on the concept of health behaviours as problematic, even outdated. Several contributors argue for a reinterpretation of the term. A significant critique of 'health behaviour' is presented that has direct relevance for the outworking of health communication efforts.

9
The Politics of Health Communication and Behaviour Change

Key aims

- To expand on the neoliberal critique and further consider the implications for health communication practice
- To critically examine the concepts of governmentality and citizenship and how these relate to issues in health communication
- To present a critique of consumption and consumer discourse in health communication
- To discuss positivism and paternalism privileging an interpretative position which forefronts lay perspectives

Introduction

This chapter brings together a critical overview of the content covered thus far and will highlight what we believe are some of the key political debates in health communication, debates that are central to health promotion considered as a more radical, social endeavour. Taking a social constructionist perspective it will unpick the notion of health communication as the route to behaviour change and challenge linear assumptions that this is the primary solution for improving health outcomes. Drawing on debate around individualism, agency and structure which are linked to concepts of citizenship and governmentality, it will appraise the politics of health communication and behaviour change within the contemporary context of an increasingly neoliberal public health agenda.

Returning to the neoliberal critique

To begin this chapter we want to return to the neoliberal critique. As outlined in Chapter 1, this is a dominant theme throughout the book. Neoliberal ideology is embedded in health communication. As highlighted, it is a specific political and economic ideology based on the individualization thesis which emphasizes personal freedom, individual control and positions the individual as an autonomous agent directing their own identity (Brannen and Nilsen, 2005). Neoliberal ideology has become more firmly embedded within so-called 'Western' contexts within the past two decades becoming a normative framework (Phipps, 2014). It now permeates all areas of human experience resulting in what Gill and Scharff (2011: 5) call 'a novel form of governance'. As previously stated, the gradual withdrawal of state welfare provision redirects responsibility into the individual subject (Aapola et al., 2005) within the private domain (Bell et al., 2011). This is reflected in the ideas discussed throughout the book which indicate how neoliberal notions of individualism, control and choice, possibility, self-invention and creation have become imbued in public health, health promotion and health communication discourse. We argue that these ideas are problematic in terms of their individualistic nature; however, Peterson and Lupton (1996: 176) argue that this may actually have an appeal to the late modern subject since such ideas 'privilege the notion of autonomous individuality'. Specific to the sphere of health, processes of individualization can be seen to be reinforced by current political ideologies which emphasize responsibility and self-determinism. We are, however, highly critical of neoliberalism and the dominance that neoliberal politics has in modern societies. The rhetoric of contemporary public health and health promotion, and the subsequent outworking of this through health communication, we would argue, focuses on neoliberal individualism and positions responsibility for health at the individual level. Individual health practices have become politicized and are increasingly part of the public rather than private domain.

The seductive allure of the independent neoliberal subject is a smoke-screen for operations of power in less visible spheres. Notions of choice, free will and personal control are peddled by neoliberal agendas and reinforced through health communication efforts, yet the *actual* control that many people have is very limited. Much of our health practices are defined and constrained by things that lie outside our (conscious and subconscious control). As Ayo (2012) points out, many choices at an individual level are constrained by social and structural factors. Barriers to authentic (or real) choice exist in societal structures such as class, gender, race and politics limiting the choices available to us. Structure and agency are inextricably linked (Measham and Shiner, 2009). When the concept of 'choice' becomes conflated with the notion of agency we neglect to consider the role that social privilege has to play simplistically positioning everyone on an equal footing. But this is not the case. Put simply, some people are able to exercise more choice than others according to the power which society ascribes to them through different structures and the resources that they have access to (Phipps, 2014). By way of example, a significant amount of research has been done into the use of insecticide treated nets (ITNs) for malaria prevention. Undoubtedly using an ITN protects people from being bitten by mosquitoes which is an important prevention strategy particularly for pregnant women and children under five years of age who are especially vulnerable to infection. But health communication efforts focus on promoting uptake and usage of ITNs often neglecting to address structural and environmental factors that impact on these such as patriarchal dominance at a household level whereby male members of the family are prioritized, lack of vector-control measures and living in poverty which leads, for example, to ITNs being used for other purposes such as being made into fishing-nets in order to secure a meal.

Health promotion's seminal document, The Ottawa Charter (WHO, 1986), recognizes the impact of our wider environment on health – that is our social, political, physical and global environments. More recently the body of work led by Sir Michael Marmot across Europe and beyond has reinforced the role that social determinants play in the creation of health. Yet still health policy tends to focus more at the individual level overemphasizing the power we have to control our health. Health communication methods appear to consistently reinforce this neoliberal discourse and the body subsequently becomes the site at which health is managed (Robertson, 2006).

As stated, responsibility for health is put onto the individual. This draws attention away from government and social responsibility for health (Room, 2011) providing a distraction from the wider, structural factors that impact on health, factors which lie outside individual control and which require action beyond an individual level (Kickbusch, 2007). This emphasizes dominant ideas of individual responsibility for health which are rooted in individualistic (Wilkinson, 2006) and neoliberal ideology (Crawshaw, 2012). For example, the focus on 'risky' individual behaviours removes government responsibility for health (in terms of tackling health inequalities for example). Critics such as Bell et al. (2011) have concerns about the focus on risky practices at an individual level in terms of how health professional rhetoric may encourage the adoption of a victim-blaming, 'self-inflicted' position that detracts from addressing structural health inequalities. This reductionist emphasis inevitably leads to attribution of blame and the creation of stigmatized identities which, in turn, leads to greater marginalization of certain groups within society. The example of obesity illustrates this. Significant psychological harm can result from focusing on obese and overweight people in health communication interventions (Graham and Edwards, 2013).

We would argue that the dominant political agenda in a 'Western' context can reasonably be described as 'anti-health promotion' particularly when we return to the radical roots of health promotion. More radical analyses of structure, such as those offered by Marxist, feminist and socialist theory, are completely lost within a neoliberal agenda. Rather, the majority of contemporary health communication calls for self-control, self-regulation and responsible citizenship (Bunton, 2006) while recognition that wider, structural factors play a major part in health outcomes is often lacking. Several critics highlight the neglect of such factors in the focus on individual behaviour (i.e. Robertson, 2006). From a critical perspective we should recognize and question this while taking into account what is achievable through individual efforts.

Implication for Practice 1

Consider the practices that you engage in and what the 'silent' politics are of the methods you use. If we are working in ways that promote the more radical nature of health promotion we need to design health communication interventions that tackle the social determinants of health at environmental and policy levels rather than those that focus purely on changes at an individual level.

Governmentality and citizenship

We now turn our attention to ideas around governmentality and citizenship which are linked to the prior discussion about neoliberalism. Governmentality theory (Foucault, 1980) is concerned with power, specifically how neoliberal modern societies control and organize people via subversive means in which individuals voluntarily participate (Crawshaw, 2012). Governmentality is centrally to do with the production of knowledge, structures of power in social processes and the constitution of subjectivity. Individualistic notions of the neoliberal subject link to ideas about governmentality (Lemke, 2007). A governmentality perspective highlights, as Crawford (2006) and Rich and Evans (2008) do, self-monitoring and personal responsibility for health as the requirement for the 'good' citizen.

For Foucault, governmentality is inextricably linked with modernity and neoliberalism and the emphasis on the individual rather than the state (Foucault, 1980). Foucault charts historical changes in the way power is exercised noting a significant shift from penalty to surveillance which took place in the eighteenth and early nineteenth centuries (Foucault, 1980; Gordon, 1980). According to Foucault this is the point in time when the mechanisms of power became more 'capillary, reaching into the very grain of individuals, touching their bodies and inserting itself into their action and attitudes, their discourse, learning processes and everyday lives' (Foucault, 1980: 112). The exercise of power became subsumed within the social body and within individual subjects (Martin, 1988). Power in health communication operates on individuals through mechanisms of control and scientific 'truths' about health and health behaviours. This is where critiques of health communication can be levelled – as a mechanism of expertise in the administration and regulation of populations (Rose and Miller, 2010).

As discussed, health promotion and public health in the postmodern era are characterized by individual responsibility. Health communication efforts reflect this. The neoliberal focus on individual responsibility (Rose, 2000) results in the requirement to strive for health (Arnoldi, 2009). There are now a set of lifestyle behaviours which are held up as being evidence of good citizenship in relation to health – ways in which we *should be* behaving (Nettleton, 2006). There is a correct or right way of *doing* health (Moore, 2010) prescribed by experts based on scientific knowledge. This becomes a moral code against which all health practices and behaviours are compared and either found to be condoned or condemned. The extent of the condemnation reflects the moral tone of a particular historical and social context. In contemporary times great attention is being paid to practices such as alcohol use, smoking, sedentary lifestyles and dietary choices for example. There is a moral obligation to take part in certain health practices in order to attain and maintain status as 'good citizens' (Peterson et al., 2010). Notably, as Joyce (2001: 598) asserts, contemporary neoliberal health policy is 'predicated on individuals taking responsibility for their own health'. Drawing on a feminist perspective it is also noteworthy that, as Moore (2008: 273) points out, 'the healthy citizen, as it is conceived of in government policy and the culture more generally is almost certainly a feminine one'.

Foucault's (1997) notion of technologies of the self is also relevant here. These refer to practices of self-discipline or 'regulatory practices' which are, in terms of this discussion, attempts to engage in lifestyles and health behaviours as prescribed by experts through health communication efforts (Ayo, 2012). Good citizenship requires the achievement of health through healthy practices and the pursuit of health which, in turn, requires disciplining the self (Peterson et al., 2010). According to Peterson and Lupton (1996) the practice of self-discipline becomes participation in healthy citizenship (re) emphasizing state concern with self-surveillance (Adkins, 2002). Through health communication individuals are exhorted and/or directed to engage in certain practices. O'Hara et al. (2015) illustrate this in what they refer to as the 'war on obesity'. O'Hara et al. (2015) undertook a critical discourse analysis on two social marketing campaigns in Australia focusing on constructions of power in the language used within the campaigns. They note the underpinning paternalistic values and assumptions within these including individualistic blaming, alarmism and moral imperatives to action. This is all evident in the way certain words are used. For example, words that instruct are used to imply authority ('individuals must take responsibility for their own health'). Certain words are also used to imply truth or certainty deriving from expert knowledge (i.e. 'obesity is caused by an imbalance of energy intake').

Shilling (1993) argues that modernity has facilitated an increase in the control exerted over bodies by institutions such as medicine (and, we would argue, public health, health promotion and health communication) in place of the reduction of the power of religion or sovereignty to define and regulate. Crawshaw (2012) points out that recent public health strategy such as social marketing for health depends on regimes of individual self-governance (for example, through diet, exercise and self-regulating alcohol consumption). This is in stark contrast to other approaches to promoting public health such as through addressing structural inequalities or through community empowerment strategies which fit more with the more radical roots of health promotion as outlined in Chapter 1.

The symbolic power of the healthy lifestyle is noted by Korp (2008: 23) who argues that 'the healthy lifestyle is always a representation of the lifestyle of a specific group in society, constructed and expressed as means of social distinction in specific fields of power'. In addition, the governance of the self is a requirement of contemporary public health and health promotion expressed through health communication messages (Peterson et al., 2010) and the body becomes the 'site of control and change through lifestyle directives' (Watson et al., 1996: 161). Power is therefore exercised through the modern day rhetoric of public health and health promotion discourse (Lupton, 2003) perpetuating the 'taken for granted authority of institutions' (Cregan, 2006: 44) and focusing on what people do (their practices and behaviours) (Shoveller and Johnson, 2006).

Normative ideas about good citizenship in terms of health are socially prescribed and defined through the power of medicine, public health and health promotion (based on expert, scientific knowledge). These are reinforced and (re)inscribed through health communication. We view this as problematic because, as Wiggins (2008: 24) contends, constructions of power are used to 'pathologize, marginalize and otherwise hold people accountable for their everyday practices'. Contemporary health and citizenship discourse are imbued with capitalist notions of consumption. Linked to this is the whole area of consumer discourse. These ideas are critically considered in the next section of this chapter.

A critique of consumption and consumer discourse in health communication

It is also necessary to consider the relationship between health and consumption or the notion of the 'consumer' and the ways in which these permeate health communication. We are critical of consumer and/or consumption discourse as linked to neoliberal and capitalist agendas and see this as subsumed/imbued in contemporary health communication. There are clear links here with the discussion about social marketing in Chapter 6. Discourses around health construct health as something which can or might be controlled by individuals through their behavioural choices. Taking risks in health becomes about making a choice (Alaszewski and Burgess, 2007) which is linked to notions of consumption and consumer choice (Harris, 2005). Specifically, the commercialization of health constructs people as 'health consumers who may consume healthy lifestyles'

(Nettleton, 2006: 47) or, indeed, unhealthy behaviours. Those that do not conform to healthy behaviours such as maintaining a 'normal' weight are cast as social failures and subject to socially sanctioned public condemnation. 'Success is measured by individual's capacity for self-care via the market, and those who do not achieve their potential are viewed as failures rather than as victims of oppressive social structures' (Phipps, 2014: 11). Never is this more apparent than in the stigmatization of the obese.

Crawford (2006) argues that capitalism both creates (and requires) a modern subject who firstly *works*, and secondly *consumes* in leisure and for pleasure. Both are necessary for capitalist society to be sustainable. There are many contributors to social scientific perspectives on health who use the concept of 'consumption' in relation to lifestyle choices and behaviours or practices (see, for example, Crawford, 2006 and Nettleton, 2006). The consumption of health is promoted by messages, for example, that overtly or covertly suggest pursuit of the 'perfect' body (slim, taut and toned). From a gendered perspective, Robertson and Williams (2010) are critical of health communication interventions and messages aimed at obese and overweight men that reproduce hegemonic masculinities such as the muscular physique.

Hart and Carter (2000) contend that there are well established patterns between certain health risks and individual behaviours of consumption (specifically citing smoking and drinking). However, as Heading (2008) notes, patterns of consumption are complex. 'For a successful consumer culture, desire must be channelled towards commodities, to make them objects of desire, regardless of intrinsic value' (Fox, 2012: 189). Health is, more and more, a target for mass consumption. It is marketed through communication strategies that promote, for example, self-management. As consumers we consciously and unconsciously buy into ideas about healthism reinforced by public health campaigns which emphasize lifestyle factors as causative agents in ill-health and disease (Bendelow, 2009). In Romania the increased use of the language of consumerism in reforms of the healthcare system has been criticized by Lanole et al. (2014: 388) for 'inspiring us to view health as just another simple commodity'.

Crawford (2000: 228) argues that, with regard to what are perceived as unhealthy behaviours, consumption is linked to a sense of deprivation juxtaposed with 'freedom to indulge'. Certainly the construction of certain types of unhealthy behaviours as more socially acceptable (less deviant) than others appears to demonstrate this. Health is also about a careful balance which requires discipline and self-control, some degree of indulgence ('letting go') but within a highly disciplined framework in order to be acceptable. Crawford's (2006: 412) conceptualization of modern capitalism in which production ('*work ethic*') and consumerism ('*pleasure ethic*') feature is useful here. Although there is more recent attention being paid to the importance of 'pleasure', it is a concept that is often missing in health communication strategies as Winter et al. (2013) point out in relation to health communication campaigns designed to reduce the incidence of hepatitis C in Australia in people who inject drugs. Among other things Winter et al. (2013) therefore recommend the acknowledgement of 'the pleasurable aspects of drug use and how emotion may influence drug use practices and decision-making' in health education materials (p. 521). Discourse around control and release in health practices draws on the notion that a little bit of release at times actually does you good (is 'healthy') (Crawford, 2006; Robertson, 2006). Unhealthy practices are reframed as healthy, as a means of coping with adversity (Smith, 2002); or a form of stress release (Harrison et al., 2011). Thus engaging in 'unhealthy' practices may actually be sanctioned and legitimized for some people in some circumstances.

Finally, in relation to consumption, we need to briefly consider the *content* of health communication messages in terms of the onus placed on the intended audience. The changing nature of knowledge (and its proliferation) requires that the recipients of health information are informed, discerning and necessarily critical. Faced with contradictory advice from numerous sources it is increasingly difficult for 'health consumers' to make informed decisions about health practices. Health information can be impenetrable, unrealistic or simply appear to be irrelevant. That is not to position lay audiences as passive and without agency, however; rather we seek to highlight the plethora of health information that is 'out there' and the challenges involved in negotiating it. These issues are discussed in greater critical depth later in this chapter and elsewhere in this book – see Chapters 5 and 8.

Implication for Practice 2

It is worth acknowledging the pleasure and happiness that people get from doing things which are labelled 'bad, harmful or risky' for health. There is the potential to reconsider how we design health communication messages in order to incorporate ideas that draw on pleasure, well-being and happiness.

Privileging interpretivist perspectives

The principles, values and practices of health promotion tie it to a social justice agenda and a commitment to tackling health inequalities using methods that are ethical and which empower. As we have already outlined, ethical and empowering practices are primarily characterized by a genuine concern for people's welfare and a willingness to enter into dialogue to commune with others (Buber, 2004; Dewey, 1997, 2008; Friere, 1972). Integral to this is the democratic process through which questions about the hidden nature of social reality are critically explored, creating a dynamic educative experience where people move from the personal (their own subjective truths) to the political (universal truths). As intended, critical dialogue reveals how inequalities are structured and reproduced, but the process also uncovers how knowledge itself is socially structured and controlled. This concept of knowledge provides the theoretical foundations for health promotion and rather crucially informs its interventions where engagement and participation are considered key. Thus, active involvement from communities to elicit their voice is integral to every aspect of health promotion work, including evaluation and research (Tones, 1999). Inviting people to participate as co-workers in evaluation and research offers further opportunities to extend the 'experiential continuum' (Dewey, 1997) so that professionals and lay people can continue to reflect critically about their shared experience and learn from it. Such opportunities for growth should necessarily include learning new skills, meeting people and, over time, building networks in the community to accrue greater social capital – an essential prerequisite for nurturing agency.

Participatory inquiry is therefore essential, not just because it is a constituent of empowerment but because its inclusive, often innovative, qualitative methods are able to interest 'heterogeneous communities' whose engagement renders a form of knowledge that is 'coherent with reality' (Mantoura and Potvin, 2012). Realist perspectives are vitally important to the health promoter as they give valuable insights into people's experiences from which professionals are often removed (Tengland, 2012). Giving a voice to marginalized groups in this way is empowering – as is the discovery about knowledge, 'engendering in lay agents a sceptical approach to all authority claims' (Potter, 1998).

However, Cruickshank (2012), Burr (2003) and Potter (2003) point out an inherent contradiction at work because although interpretivist approaches engage with the marginalized effectively – enabling them to share their individual personal truths – it can empower them no further as it considers *all* such subjective truths to be of equal worth. This philosophical position ultimately conflates truth claims with personal perspectives – a position that is deeply problematic for the morally obligated, action-oriented discipline of health promotion, because in denying the existence of truth claims (i.e. poverty exists because of an unequal distribution of wealth) it also takes away the justification to challenge or take action. Realist-social constructionists counter this critique claiming truth *can* be attained using interpretivism *if* the knowledge that is co-produced is debated and negotiated (Mantoura and Potvin, 2012). This returns us to the Freirean concept of socially constructed knowledge alluded to earlier, whereby individual personal concerns (subjective truths) develop to include collective political perspectives (universal truths) through critical dialogue and *conscientization*.

Critiquing positivism

In recent years there has been growing criticism of the scientific method in health promotion (Raphael, 2000; Polanyi et al., 2005; Tannahill, 2008), highlighting the fundamental unsuitability of positivist concepts of knowledge to assess interventions that typically involve 'complex multi-layered, multifactorial programmes often delivered in a cumulative fashion over a long period of time' (Tones, 1999: 228). The 'scientific method' (Hennink et al., 2011) uses quantitative methods of inquiry which require tangible evidence of a cause and effect relationship. This is predicated on the empiricist belief that knowledge is derived via the senses and so, unsurprisingly, it emphasizes the importance of observable repeated regularities as proof of such a relationship. However, as its critics point out, this does not reflect what happens in the social world where the relationship between cause and effect is often unobservable and extremely complex to fathom. Acknowledging the shortcomings of the scientific method more than twenty years ago, WHO concluded, 'evaluators need to use a wide range of qualitative and qualitative methods that extend beyond the narrow perimeters of randomized controlled trials' (WHO, 1998: 11).

Although the use of qualitative, interpretivist methods of inquiry has increased within health promotion today, powerful positivist notes still linger in public health where health promoters are often located. According to Tones (1999) this continuing influence exists because of the powerful 'hegemony of medicine in relation to "satellite" occupations and disciplines' – such as health promotion. While this is undeniable, evidence does suggest that until recently public health professionals were engaging more with participatory forms of inquiry. Indeed, there might have been a cultural shift away from the clinical, positivist model had it not been for the transformative effect of neoliberal policies on health authorities, public health departments and healthcare industries (Raphael, 2008). In the UK, these policies have promoted a business orientation within publicly funded health services and introduced managerialist practices that have given rise to an audit culture – a culture which essentially quantifies all actions as transactions. Thus, health promotion expenditure (which now has to be identified in advance) is itemized and accounted for using specialist software programmes, and once having been valued in monetary terms, health promotion interventions are then valued summatively for efficacy by being directly, and unproblematically, linked to health outcomes. In this climate, health promotion reverts to being 'expert-driven, authoritarian and disempowering' (Davies and Macdonald, 1998: 209) with a focus on short-term behaviour change as a tangible way of communicating effectiveness and value for money. Inevitably this is how the majority of health communication efforts also manifest.

Post-positivism and the critical realist approach

Given the current constraints that hinder a more radical interpretation of health promotion as a social endeavour a new social theory for health promotion, and therefore health communication, is required; one that (a) reflects the real messiness of life; (b) supports the ideals and activities of emancipatory praxis; (c) encourages individual and collective autonomy; and (d) illuminates the structure–agency relationship to shed light upon the complex causes and effects within the *social world*. Archer's theory of human agency does just this (Archer, 1995, 2000). Avoiding both upward conflationary theories which overplay the power of the individual *and* downward conflationary theories that present people as the victims of circumstance, Archer provides a critical realist account of how, over time and under certain conditions, people can become powerful enough to effect transformations at all levels. This is an emancipatory social theory that is perfectly suited to radical health promotion and health communication praxis, and reveals to the practitioner the contingent requirements for agency – arguably *the* essential kernel of empowerment and the essence of health promotion. This leads us to consider the centrality of the lay perspective in health communication.

The importance of lay perspectives

Involving the public (lay people) in health matters is seen as an accepted principle in contemporary society in many contexts. It is recognized, at least in terms of winning the moral argument, that the public should be active partners in service provision rather than passive recipients of paternalistic professional actions (Taylor, 2007). The debate is, however, about *how* and *at what level* they are involved within a bio-medical and professional dominated society where the expert knowledge is privileged. Lay people have always been informal carers at home, often hidden and unrecognized (Parker, 1990). However, involving lay people at a policy level, in research and in decision-making within service delivery has been rather tokenistic and often about reactive consultation with very short deadlines for feedback. In the UK attempts to recognize lay perspectives at a Governmental level can be seen in advisory documents The Expert Patient Programme in Long Term Illness Management (DH, 2001) and, in the last few years, the recommendations of 'co-production' in Public Service delivery during the second half of the New Labour Government with ideas such as 'personal budgets' and self-directed support, carried forward under the Coalition Government (Boyle et al., 2010).

User involvement can be a challenge to the expertise of the professionals, as seen in Prior's (2003) paper on lay knowledge and lay experts in medicine where she challenged the 'expertise' of lay people and questioned whether the life experience of lay people on its own can equate to the understanding of the technical complexities of disease causation, its consequences or its management. The rhetoric of involvement can also conceal an unwillingness on the part of professionals to cede real power – indicative perhaps of a much wider trend. Using an example of smoking cessation intervention, Springett (2007) examined the contribution of lay knowledge in informing health-promotion practices. Lay expertise can be seen as important at the delivery stage, rather than having any value in the development of interventions. There are many other studies which focus on lay perspectives on health and illness. For example, Aubel et al. (2004)

on Senegalese grandmothers promoting maternal and child nutrition practice; Emslie (2005) on men and women's knowledge of coronary heart disease and Swami et al. (2009) about lay perspectives of health and illness. The competing paradigms of knowledge creation in evidence-based practice that prefer the 'expert' or scientific, generalizable knowledge can decontextualize knowledge by ignoring everyday reality and experience. Older people from BME communities, commenting on a review of UK-based research about their lives, said they had often been involved in these projects in the 1990s (Butt and O'Neil, 2004). However, they also reported that researchers had usually asked the wrong research questions then and were still asking the wrong questions at the time the paper was published.

In relation to communicating health messages, information is usually seen as flowing one-way from health experts to lay people (Lee and Garvin, 2003). Lay perspectives are rarely taken into account. People's understanding of health and illness depends on the context of their experience in life, socially and culturally, and it relates to time and space (Popay et al., 1998). Lay knowledge about health is completely different from that of the positivistic, reductive medical profession. People's own views about their own health can be dismissed as subjective and personal. However there are profound issues of ontology, epistemology and paradigm which challenge professionalized knowledge. For example, disabled people created the Social Model of Disability to challenge the medicalized views of their lives in society as a whole and among medical 'experts' in particular (Carson, 2009). The need to challenge professionalized knowledge stretches far beyond disabled people versus professionalized knowledge, however and includes parallel challenges from feminists, older people and the Civil Rights movement in the USA and beyond (Branfield and Beresford, 2006). It is important, in terms of equity but also in terms of practicality, that people take actions and make decisions about their health choices and having control of their own health based on their knowledge. Lay knowledge provides meanings to events which orientate actions (Popay et al., 1998). This is crucial to health communication. Often people's own constructions of health and multiple realities is placed at the periphery rather than in the mainstream of public health and wider aspects of health (Branfield and Beresford, 2006).

Lay involvement is both about involving people in their own individual experiences but also collectively in helping to shape policy and practice responses (Carter and Beresford, 2000). Popay et al. (1998) argued for a narrative form of research in health and social inequalities that helps practitioners and policy makers gain a deeper understanding of health variations based on people's social context and social structure, so that actions can be more meaningful. The upstream approach to health and the social determinants of health have brought a wider understanding of health and what constitute public health actions within the Social Model of Health. Health is defined by much more than objective measurable outcomes. The understanding of people's lived experience within their own social context in mainstream public health is still far from satisfactory although significant strides are being made in some contexts (South et al., 2013).

Barriers in user involvement in social research and in policy and decision-making process can result in lay people being marginalized by professionals in partnership working (Branfield and Beresford, 2006; Forrest et al., 2013). The power of biomedical discourse in defining the terms of engagement is a major barrier in user involvement. Taylor (2007) identified four approaches to promoting lay contributions to public health – the *consumerist approach* where lay people are being consulted as consumer of services; the *representative approach* where lay people sit on committees as representatives for the public; the *interest group approach* where lay people form small interest groups on a particular cause and the *network approach* where health professionals can find out about the lived experiences of communities through networking with them. We would argue that this can only work when issues of power among lay populations are addressed. Indeed, some service users argue that, unless such issues are addressed, some forms of participation can be a waste of time or even harmfully manipulative (Branfield and Beresford, 2006). Most lay people are often powerless in influencing any actions, particularly for those who are not confident in challenging hierarchical expertise, and when they are too overwhelmed by the business of surviving and making ends meet.

Arnstein's (1969) ladder of citizen participation illustrates levels of participation as rungs on a ladder, from the lowest rung of manipulation to the highest rung of citizen control. In health communication efforts we are often, at worst, operating in a persuasive and manipulative manner. At best we should be working with people enabling true empowerment control. Partnership working is increasingly encouraged in public health. The challenge lie in how people are involved and at what level power is relinquished to people – the 'power over' moving to 'power with' (Laverack, 2013), so that people are empowered and lay voices are heard and taken seriously. Indeed, there is compelling evidence that sharing power can be a 'win-win' for lay people and professional people alike (Forrest et al., 2013). Green et al.'s (2015) participation and the empowerment gradient is a useful way to illustrate when people are being excluded, manipulated or coerced into following instruction. This is relative powerlessness. When participation increases, where people have control, are supported to participate and are involved in decision-making, they can be empowered. In terms of health communication, decisions about sustainable behaviour change need to be made by people themselves based on their choices and their circumstances. The development of healthy public policies and health promotion interventions within organizations as well as at government level should be made with full participation at decision-making level for individuals and also for communities. It is also important to recognize and tackle the social, economic, environmental *and* political structural barriers that individuals and communities face in realizing this.

Implication for Practice 3
Empowerment means encouraging real participation, valuing lay perspectives in decision-making, perhaps relinquishing some of the power that we have as 'experts' in order to maximize empowerment for those whom we work with.

Implication for Practice 4
Practice in health communication needs to be critically considered in the context of the points raised in this chapter. It is worth questioning what we do and why. We should be reflecting on whether we promote a paternalistic, top-down agenda which privileges expert opinion and quantifiable outcomes. We should be considering how we can maximize empowerment and transformation and how we create opportunities for lay voices to be heard, listened to and acted upon.

Summary of key points

This chapter has discussed a number of key issues related to the politics of health communication. Specifically it has:

- expanded upon the neoliberal critique and further considered the implications for health communication practice

- examined the concepts of governmentality and citizenship and how these relate to issues in health communication
- presented a critique of consumption and consumer discourse in health communication
- critiqued positivism and paternalism privileging an interpretative position which forefronts lay perspectives

---

Reflection 1 – It is worth considering your own values and personal political persuasion. Where do you sit on the individual responsibility versus state responsibility for health continuum and why? Are you inclined sometimes to blame people for the situation they find themselves in? To what extent is this justifiable? Acknowledging your own position will help to inform your practice.

Reflection 2 – You may wish to read more about governmentality and citizenship. Do you agree that we are living in a world of increased surveillance? What implications may this have for health communication? The rise of self-monitoring of health through digital devices is an interesting area that you may want to explore further.

Reflection 3 – Do you seek out and encourage user involvement in deciding and designing health communication strategies? How much power do you have? Do you involve the people you work with in the decision-making process? How? Is it enough? Who sets the agenda? Is any of the budget set aside for lay people to get training? When was the last time a meeting included lay voices?

Reflection 4 – How much power do you have in terms of influencing policies in your organization or at a local, regional and national governmental level? Do you have a voice? How and where? If you are not being 'heard' how can you make this happen?

Further reading

Ayo, N. (2012) Understanding health promotion in a neoliberal climate and the making of health conscious citizens. *Critical Public Health*, 22, 99–105.
This paper expands on some of the key arguments presented in this chapter and critically considers the role of contemporary health promotion in the creation of neoliberal subjects striving for health.
Lupton, D. (2016) *The Quantified Self.* Cambridge: Polity.

This book considers the contemporary phenomenon of self-tracking and personal surveillance practices exploring the social, cultural and political dimensions of these.

South, J., White, J. and Gamsu, M. (2013) *People-Centred Public Health*. Bristol: Policy Press.

Drawing on a major piece of research about lay engagement this book focuses on how ordinary people can be involved in health improvement. It uses case studies and real-life examples throughout.

10
Looking to the Future

In *Health Communication: Theoretical and Critical Perspectives* we have sought to provide a more critical perspective on the assumptions, ideologies and values underpinning well-rehearsed approaches in health communication. In the first part of this book we outlined what we see as the three key disciplinary perspectives that are key to health communication: education, communication and psychology. We discussed and critiqued a range of theory with reference to international research literature throughout. In the second part of the book we considered a number of contemporary areas in health communication: methods and media, social marketing and health literacy. In the third part of the book we focused on some of the broader challenges in health communication. In this final chapter we consider what some of the future challenges in health communication might be. This chapter therefore brings the book to a close and suggests some of the challenges that face us within a rapidly changing world. It considers some of the possible directions for communication for health promotion within the context of huge advances in information communication technology, globalization and changes in human interaction.

In a Bulletin of the World Health Organization published in 2009, Rimal and Lapkinski argued that health communication was of growing importance. They based this observation on the fact that, for the first time, health communication was allocated a chapter in the United States of America's Healthy People 2010 Objectives. However, the central thrust of this was, perhaps unsurprisingly, health behaviours. Rimal and Lapkinski (2009) took an optimistic stance on the potential of health communication efforts as a means to improve and save lives contending that we are living in a time where 'many of the threats to global public health (through diseases and environmental calamities) are rooted in human behaviour' (p. 247). This argument has some merit and provides the underpinnings for neoliberal approaches to promoting public health. However, we have, in this book, expounded upon some of the significant limitations of relying solely on such approaches despite the persuasive nature of the arguments given in support of them. Ethical concerns in health communication are a key theme that runs through this book. We need to take care, in health communication practice, to avoid adverse effects at an individual and societal level such as stigmatizing certain people (Loss and Nagel, 2009) and instead capitalize on the potential of health communication to empower, transform and emancipate.

More recently the importance of health communication was reiterated in the European context by a technical report published by the European Centre for Disease Prevention and Control entitled 'Health communication and its role in the prevention and control of communicable disease in Europe: Current evidence, practice and future developments' (Sixsmith et al., 2014). Again, the document highlights the role of health communication in addressing the continuing and growing threat of communicable diseases in public health in Europe. Drawing on expertise from each of the thirty European Union and EEA countries the report identifies a number of challenges and priorities including that most of the evidence in health communication originates from North America and that there is 'a lack of knowledge on how to use health communication to effectively engage and improve health outcomes for hard-to-reach groups' (p. 2). The report also noted that there was inconsistency across Europe in terms of capacity for health communication producing variability in practice. This, as we know, can and does lead to greater health inequality. In short, the report suggested a number of things to improve health communication efforts which have resonance with the arguments put forward in this book including the incorporation of health communication activities into health policy and strategy, enhanced collaborative working and greater coordination. Significantly, the report highlights 'the importance of partnerships with community groups (reflecting) a new paradigm of citizen-centred health communication with the identification of the inclusion of citizen stakeholders as active partners in health communication endeavours . . .' (Sixsmith et al., 2014: 3).

Challenging the mechanisms of global health communication

Global health communication inextricably links health with human behaviour. The key justification for this is that the major health challenges facing the world's population are viewed as being driven, or caused by, human behaviour. Consequently efforts are directed at developing behaviour change communication interventions aimed at specific groups of people which are underpinned by the problematic assumptions challenged by the arguments in this book. This agenda is driven, at a global level, by the key players in global health that arguably promote a specific agenda based on theoretical and empirical frameworks dominated by Western ideologies. Manyozo (2012) offers an alternative theoretical framework for developing world contexts which integrates community media within health communication strengthening social capital, social infrastructure and social economy. Manyozo's (2012) rationale for suggesting an alternative approach is that 'traditional' health communication theory falls short, particularly in terms of promoting meaningful engagement and privileging indigenous knowledge. In short, this reflects a bottom-up approach in keeping with health promotion's concerns which centres on processes of community development. As Manyozo (2012) argues, the challenge then becomes about promoting community health engagement rather than telling people how they should be behaving and endorsing adherence to 'best health practices' as characterized by the dominant health communication models. The notion of 'best health practices' leads us onto another challenge in health communication, namely 'healthism'.

Crossley (2002: 1471) presents a convincing argument proposing that health is an 'intrinsically moral phenomenon'. Equating being healthy with being of good or sound moral character is a theme that recurs in discourse on health and health behaviour (Roy, 2008). Crawford (2006) uses the phrase 'healthism' for what he describes as the moralization of health. The moralizing of health is something which has been discussed extensively in the literature (Robertson, 2006), specifically around health practices and the moral imperative of responsibility for health (Bolam et al., 2003). This is evident in much of health communication discourse. Crossley (2002) argues that this has resulted in the identification of a range of practices which are deemed unhealthy and subsequently equate to being 'bad' or 'immoral' or deviant. The pursuit of health (and therefore 'sound moral character') becomes an imperative (Roy, 2008) and we become morally obligated to take part in certain health practices in order to attain and maintain status as 'good citizens' (Peterson et al., 2010). Despite these critiques we see these ideas replicated in health communication efforts around the world and the focus on trying to 'rectify' behaviour at an individual level. A review of health communication campaigns in developing countries by Sood et al. (2014) looked at forty-eight different pieces of published literature discussing developing country campaigns. The review determined that a number of different strategies were used, yet the focus was very much still at changing behaviour at an individual level perpetuating these dominant ideas.

Changing technologies: implications for health communication

We live in an increasingly connected world. Technology is changing and developing apace. The ways in which we communicate with each other and receive information is unrecognizable from two decades ago. In Chapter 5 – Methods and Media – we expound upon the use of different types of media and the potential impact, positive and negative, that these can have on health communication. Undoubtedly advances in technology have the potential to bring about significant changes to health and to be harnessed for more effective health communication. Nevertheless, there is significant debate about the potential of the internet to improve health, particularly around the provision of health information. Access to health information and the utility of it links to health literacy which we discussed in detail in Chapter 7. There are considerable advantages to using the internet for health communication including reach, relative low cost and convenience. Despite well-documented challenges such as inconsistent information and the generally high levels of literacy required there are arguments that providing health information via the internet can empower people, promote decision-making and reduce the expert/lay divide (Henwood et al., 2003; Benigeri and Pluye, 2003). However, there is also the potential for greater inequalities and social disparities linked to access to the technology required which in turn may widen health inequalities. Generally speaking, the poorest in society have less access and are more likely to be in greatest need (Sinden and Wister, 2008). In addition to differences in access according to income there are differences in terms of age. Consequently younger, more wealthy people tend to benefit more resulting in what is known as 'the digital divide' (Sinden and Wister, 2008). The digital divide also refers to discrepancies in internet access whereby typically, on a global level, internet use is more likely in higher income and educated populations. In addition, across all country contexts more men than women tend to use technology and there is a divide between internet/technology access for rural and urban populations (Bam and Girase, 2015). Research into eHealth strategies in Bangladesh shows how progress is slowed by limited bandwidth and the high cost of infrastructure support systems and software development (Shariful Islam and Tabassum, 2015). This is often an issue in resource-poor settings.

We can appreciate, however, the potential of information communication and technology in relatively resource-poor settings particularly with young people. In the South Asian context, Bam and Girase (2015) argue that there are numerous benefits to using newer technologies such as mobile devices in tackling issues in adolescent sexual health education including low cost, increased access to remote populations, efficiency and flexibility. Talking about m- and e-technologies and young people Bam and Girase (2015) argue that 'the future potential is likely to be something mobile, digital and alive that can connect adolescents with various provision' (p. 5). Social media has enormous potential to improve health. Nevertheless, we need to be aware that (particularly in the context of developing countries) disparity often exists in accessibility and use (Anand et al., 2013).

A new paradigm – thinking 'social theories of practice'

In Chapter 4 – Psychological Theory – we are critical of the notion of 'health behaviour' and debate the merits of using terms such as 'social practices' instead. As we write this final chapter a new idea is emerging which is worth brief reference here. In the context of trying to address a number of behavioural factors related to non-communicable diseases Blue et al. (2016) argue for a total paradigmatic shift. They contrast the individualistic approaches to behaviour change (read 'health communication') which dominate the academic research literature with action at structural levels to address health inequalities and the social determinants of health. They suggest an alternative paradigm as the way forward; one that denotes a significant shift in conceptual understanding. That is, the use of *social theories of practice*, specifically focusing on the lifecourse and how the material and symbolic elements of certain practices are comprised and change over time (Blue et al., 2016). Using smoking as an example they argue the case for this approach noting how there are often strong relations between smoking and other practices such as socializing, leisure and alcohol use. Using such an approach, they argue, would promote understanding of processes of change. Consequently Blue et al. (2016: 45) contend that 'if we want to know how social practices develop over time, or what can be done to change them, it makes little sense to ask what motivates or constrains individuals'. They challenge the 'dominance and power of, on the one hand, the individualistic behavioural paradigm, and, on the other, the wider determinants approach' (46) arguing instead that the way in which behaviour change is tackled needs to be rethought. They do acknowledge that this would not be easy, however, since it 'calls for a major change in the theoretical foundation of public health policy and for corresponding forms of methodological inventiveness and ingenuity' (47). For further explication please see Blue et al. (2016).

Critical analysis in health communication

One of the key intentions in this book, in keeping with a health promotion perspective, has been to bring issues of power and empowerment to the fore. We therefore advocate for the use of critical perspectives and techniques to highlight and challenge power and ideology in health communication. One of the ways in which this can be achieved is by critically analysing discourse and the way in which discursive practices serve to maintain and promote structures of power within society. If we can identify 'power interests buried within texts (and talk)' (O'Hara et al., 2015: 1) it paves the way for the questioning and disruption of these. By way of example O'Hara et al. (2015) used Critical Discourse Analysis to analyse a weight-focused social marketing campaign in Australia. They critiqued the paternalistic, individualistic, moralistic and coercive nature of the campaign arguing that it served to stigmatize 'fat people' yet make them invisible at the same time. O'Hara et al. (2015) concluded by calling for public health efforts to be aware of the unintended yet harmful effects that such campaigns can result in. This paper illustrates the key focus of the obesity 'agenda' in general which highlights some of the problematic approaches in health communication that we have expounded upon in this book – namely the lack of attention to addressing structural factors such as social, environmental and economic issues. Being critical of the neoliberal agenda and the individualist, deterministic focus of it we would argue that health communication efforts should provoke action at political and structural levels in addressing contemporary public health concerns. One such approach would be to tackle our 'obesogenic' environment (Chaput et al., 2011).

A challenge to competency frameworks

Sixsmith et al. (2014) define health communication competencies as 'the combination of the essential knowledge, abilities, skills and values necessary for the practice of health communication' (p. 4), a definition they have adapted from Dempsey et al. (2011). As should be evident by now, we have used an approach within this book which moves away from defining and discussing a set of competencies for health communication. Although we have suggested implications for practice, and sometimes policy, it has not been our intention to provide a 'how-to' guide for health communication. Other books aim to provide this. Rather, we set out to produce a critical take on much of the received wisdom that is taken for granted in health communication drawing on broader perspectives and critiquing the underpinning political and structural dimensions. Nevertheless, using a positivist framework, considerable efforts have been put into developing health promotion competencies or standards of practice. Our arguments throughout this book provide a critique of such deterministic approaches (see Chapter 3 on Educational Theory). So, while the Galway Consensus (Barry et al., 2009), for example, may have merit in terms of providing a set of core competencies for health promotion practice we would question the basis on which this is founded. Interestingly, however, there appears to have been relatively little critique of this.

As we write this final chapter (early 2016) a review of the UK's 2008 Public Health Knowledge and Skills Framework (PHKSF) is taking place which began in spring 2015 (PHE, 2015). As a team we have taken up the opportunity to comment on this review in a widespread consultancy exercise. We approached this, primarily, from an academic perspective. Within the context of the critique about competency frameworks we offer in this chapter we view the proposed new framework as an improvement on the previous one. Health inequalities are much more centre-stage and the context is taken into account more. However, the new framework apparently tends to favour more top-down than bottom-up approaches and there is a relative lack of attention given to certain things that we would argue are crucial in improving health such as community development and participation. Unfortunately, to our minds, the new framework seems to promote expert-led *doing unto* rather than true engagement with communities or facilitating action. While the increased focus on health inequalities is laudable there does not appear to be enough content specific to tackling the social and environmental determinants of health. It remains to be seen what the final framework will actually look like; however, we are optimistic that our views, and others of similar minds, will be taken into account in the final outcome.

Towards the future in health communication

It is difficult to predict with any certainty what the future holds in terms of health communication. We have witnessed rapid changes in society at local and global levels in recent years and continue to do so. Each new day brings with it more change and more challenge. The post-modern revolution in communication and technology brings with it unparalleled potential but also paradoxical challenges. For the relatively privileged continuing globalization and technological advancement will no doubt increase individual possibilities and agency to shape their own private worlds as well as allowing them to continue to exercise their unrepresentative power in shaping the world. This is not insignificant. At the time of writing (early 2016) Oxfam International estimated that the sixty-two richest individuals in our world have the same wealth as the poorest 3.6 billion (or nearly half the global population). That is a crazy statistic whichever way you look at it! Of course, globalization and technological advancements may also allow those with little access to wealth and privilege in any form to also shape their private worlds to some extent but this is likely to occur within a neoliberal agenda which therefore reinforces the existing hegemony.

In a world where social and economic divisions are increasing within a global political hegemony that privileges monetarism, these forces might trigger a perverse return to patriarchal localism or retrograde versions of anarchy – a rejection of neoliberal values but in a social and/or political vacuum that potentially lets in old fundamentalism. If governments world-wide fail to plan and structure their societies as well as economies together along the lines of access they will risk alienating their citizens further – citizens who already, due to the same forces mentioned previously, do not conform to any traditional notions of social cohesion or have any predictable patterns of political affinity. Unchecked, the major health outcomes of post-modernity will be around managing the casualties of war. This might be direct or indirect as we have seen in the latter part of 2015 and early months of 2016 with the vast number of refugees on the move into and across Europe. The results of such social change are not insignificant and will call for different ways of working to promote health. Increasingly we see the need to challenge the negative effects of post-modernity and the requirement to pay greater attention than ever to relatively powerless communities – those who suffer due to restricted access to the basic needs of life and who are at increased risk of poorer health in all spheres.

Final comments

In conclusion, we hope that you have enjoyed reading this book as much as we have enjoyed researching and writing it. We have all learnt a great deal along the way. We set out with the intention of challenging our readers and exposing you to new ways of thinking about things that you may have previously taken for granted and indeed, we have experienced this ourselves during this book's journey to completion. We have found it a challenge to write, rightly so for a book of this kind. One of the major issues has been trying to find literature about health communication that goes against the mainstream and challenges current understanding and practice. To this end we have drawn on a range of different perspectives, academic writing and international research to support our arguments.

At the outset, in Chapter 1, we outlined our critical theoretical position framing our interest in health communication within the wider remit of contemporary health promotion. We have therefore explicated our arguments in this book within a specific ideological, political and philosophical arena, which privileges the more radical perspectives at the core of health promotion as espoused by the values and principles underpinning it. These are worth outlining again at this point: namely empowerment, equity, tackling health inequalities, addressing the social determinants of health, privileging a social model of health, advocacy, ethical practice, participation, collaboration and upstream approaches. We have used this 'health promotion lens' to scrutinize a range of issues pertinent to contemporary health communication theory and practice. Our hope is that, in some way, engaging with the material in this book will enable you to reflect on and hopefully change your practice in health communication. We wish you every success in doing so.

References

Aapola, S., Gonick, M. and Harris, A. (2005) *Young Femininity; Girlhood, Power and Social Change*. Basingstoke: Palgrave Macmillan.

Abolfotouh, M. A. et al. (2015) Using the health belief model to predict breast self-examination among Saudi women. *BMC Public Health*, 15, 1163–75.

Abraham, C. and Sheeran, P. (2005) The health belief model. In Connor, M. and Norman, P. (eds) *Predicting Health Behaviours*. 2nd edn. Buckingham: Open University Press, pp. 28–80.

Acheson, D. (1998) *Independent Inquiry into Inequalities in Health: Recommendations*. London: Department of Health.

Adkins, L. (2002) Risk, sexuality and economy. *British Journal of Sociology*, 53, 19–40.

Ahmad, F., Hudak, P. L., Bercovitz, K., Hollenberg, E. and Levinson, W. (2006) Are physicians ready for patients with Internet-based health information? *Journal of Medical Internet Research*, 8 (3), e22.

Airhihenbuwa, C. O. and Obregon, R. (2000) A critical assessment of theories/models used in health communication for HIV/AIDS. *Journal of Health Communication*, 5, 5–15.

Ajzen, I. (1988) The theory of planned behavior. *Organizational Behavior and Human Decision Processes*, 50, 179–211.

Ajzen, I. (1992) Persuasive communication theory in social psychology: a historical perspective. In Manfredo, M. J. (ed.) *Influencing Human Behaviour: Theory and Application in Recreation and Tourism*. Champaign, IL: Sagamore Publishing, pp. 1–27.

Alaszewski, A. (2005) Risk communication: identifying the importance of social context. *Health, Risk and Society*, 7, 101–5.

Alaszewski, A. and Burgess, A. (2007) Risk, time and reason. *Health, Risk and Society*, 9, 349–58.

Alexander, S. A. C., Frohlich, K. L., Poland, B. D., Haines, R. J. and Maule, C. (2010) I'm a young student, I'm a girl . . . and for some reason they are hard on me for smoking: the role of gender and the social context for smoking behaviour. *Critical Public Health*, 20, 323–38.

Allman, P. (1988) Gramsci, Freire and Illich: their contributions to education for socialism. In Lovett, T. (ed.) *Radical Approaches to Adult Education: A Reader*. London: Routledge, pp. 85–113.

Allman, P. and Wallis, J. (1995) Challenging the postmodern condition: radical adult education for critical intelligence. In Mayo, M. and Thompson, J. (eds) *Adult Learning, Critical Intelligence and Social Change*. Leicester: National Institute of Adult Continuing Education.

Allmark, P. and Tod, A. M. (2013) Can a nudge keep you warm? Using nudges to reduce excess winter deaths: insight from the Keeping Warm in Later Life Project (KWILLT). *Journal of Public Health*, 36 (1), 111–16.

Anand, S., Gupta, M. and Kwatra, S. (2013) Social media and effective health communication. *International Journal of Social Science and Interdisciplinary Research*, 2 (8), 39–46.

Ancker, J. S., Weber, E. U. and Kukafka, R. (2011) Effects of game-like interactive graphics on risk perceptions and decisions. *Medical Decision Making*, Jan–Feb, 130–42.

Anderson, P. and Nishtar, S. (2011) Communicating the non-communicable. *Journal of Health Communication: International Perspectives*, 16, (s2), 6–12.

Andreasen, A.R. (2002) Marketing social marketing in the social change marketplace. *Journal of Public Policy Marketing*, 21 (1), 3–13.

Archer, M. S. (1995) *Realist Social Theory: The Morphogenetic Approach*. Cambridge: Cambridge University Press.

Archer, M. S. (2000) *Being Human: The Problem of Agency*. Cambridge: Cambridge University Press.

Aristotle (2004) *The Nicomachean Ethics*. London: Penguin.

Arnoldi, J. (2009) *Risk*. Cambridge: Polity.

Arnstein, S. (1969) A ladder of citizen participation. *Journal of the American Institute of Planners*, 35, 216–24.

Aschemann-Witzel, J., Perez-Cueto, F. J. A., Niedzwiedzka, B., Verbeke, W. and Bech-Larsen, T. (2012) Lessons for public health campaigns from analysing commercial food marketing success factors: a case study. *BMC Public Health*, 12, 139–50.

Atkin, C. K. and Rice, R. E. (2013) *Advances in Public Communication Campaigns*. http://www.comm.ucsb.edu/faculty/rrice/C59AtkinRice2013. pdf

Atkin, C. K. and Salmon, C. (2010) Communication campaigns. In Berger, C., Roloff, M. and Roskos-Ewoldsen, D. (eds) *Handbook of Communication Sciences*. 2nd edn. Thousand Oaks, CA: Sage, pp. 419–35.

Aubel, J., Toure, I. and Diagneb, M. (2004) Senegalese grandmothers promote improved maternal and child nutrition practices: the guardians of tradition are not averse to change. *Social Science and Medicine*, 59, 945–59.

Austen, L. (2009) The social construction of risk by young people. *Health, Risk and Society*, 11, 451–70.

Australian Social Trends (1997) *Changing Industries, Changing Jobs*. Available at http://www.abs.gov.au/

Avis, J. (2004) Workplace learning, knowledge, practice and transformation. *Journal for Critical Education Policy Studies*, 8 (2), 166–93.

Ayo, N. (2012) Understanding health promotion in a neoliberal climate and the making of health conscious citizens. *Critical Public Health*, 22, 99–105.

Backett-Milburn, K. and Wilson, S. (2000) Understanding peer education: insights from a process evaluation. *Health Education Research*, 15 (1), 5–96.

Badarudeen, S. and Sabharwal, S. (2010) Assessing readability of patient education materials: current role in orthopaedics. *Clinical Orthopaedics and Related Research*, 468 (10), 2572.

Balatti, J., Black, S. and Falk, I. (2009) *A New Social Capital Paradigm for Adult Literacy: Partnerships, Policy and Pedagogy* – Support document, NCVER (National Centre of Vocational Education Research).

Bam, K. and Girase, B. (2015) Scenario of adolescent sexual and reproductive health with opportunities for information communication and technology use in selected South Asian countries. *Health Science Journal*, 9 (42), 1–7.

Barker, K., Lowe, C. M. and Reid, M. (2006) *The Use of Mass Media Interventions for Health Care Messages About Back Pain: What Do Members of the Public Think?* Oxford, UK: Nuffield Orthopaedic Centre NHS Trust.

Baron-Epel, O., Satran, C., Cohen, V., Drach-Zehavi, A. and Hovell, M. F. (2012) Challenges for the smoking ban in Israeli pubs and bars: an analysis guided by the behavioural ecological model. *Israel Journal of Health Policy Research*, 1, 28 http:www.ijhpr.org/content/1/1/28

Barr, A., Stenhouse, C. and Henderson, P. (2001) *Caring Communities: A Challenge for Social Inclusion*. York: York Publishing Service.

Barry, M., Allegrante, J. P. and Lamarre, M. (2009) The Galway Consensus Conference: international collaboration on the development of core competencies for health promotion and health education. *Global Health Promotion*, 16 (2), 5–11.

Bauer, G. R. (2014) Incorporating intersectionality theory into population health research methodology: challenges and the potential to advance health equity. *Social Science and Medicine*, 110, 10–17.

Baum, F. (2002) *The New Public Health*. 2nd edn. Melbourne: Oxford University Press.

Baum, F. and Fisher, M. (2014) Why behavioural health promotion endures despite its failure to reduce health inequities. *Sociology of Health and Illness*, 36 (2), 213–25.

Bavarian, N. et al. (2014) Using structural equation modelling to understand prescription stimulant misuse: a test of the Theory of Triadic Influence. *Drug and Alcohol Dependence*, 138, 193–201.

Baxter, L. A. and Braithwaite, D. O. (2008) *Engaging Theories in Interpersonal Communication: Multiple Perspectives*. London: Sage.

Beauchamp, D. (1976) Public health as social justice. *Inquiry*, 13 (1), 3–14.

Bell, K., Salmon, A. and McNaughton, D. (2011) Editorial: Alcohol, tobacco, obesity and the new public health. *Critical Public Health*, 21, 1–8.

Bendelow, G. (2009) *Health, Emotion and the Body*. Cambridge: Polity.

Benigeri, M. and Pluye, P. (2003) Shortcomings of health information on the Internet. *Health Promotion International*, 18 (4), 381–6.

Bennett, A. E. (1975) *Communication Between Doctors and Patients*. Oxford: Oxford University Press.

Bennett, G. G. and Glasgow, R. E. (2009) The delivery of public health interventions via the Internet: actualizing their potential. *Annual Review of Public Health*, 30, 273–92.

Benoit, C. et al. (2014) Providers' constructions of pregnant and early parenting women who use substances. *Sociology of Health and Illness*, 36 (2), 157–62.

Benzeval, M., Bond, L., Campbell, M., Egan, M., Lorenc, T., Petticrew, M. and Popham, F. (2014) *Report: How Does Money Influence Health?* York: Joseph Rowntree Foundation.

Beresford, P., Nettle, M. and Perring, J. (2010) *Towards a Social Model of Madness and Distress*. York: Joseph Rowntree Foundation.

Beresford, P. et al. (2011) *Supporting People – Towards a Person-Centred Approach*. Bristol: Policy Press.

Beresford, P., Nettle, M. and Perring, J. (2016, forthcoming) *From Mental Illness Towards a Social Model of Madness and Distress*. London: Shaping Our Lives.

Berger, A. A. (1995) *Essentials of Mass Communication Theory*. London: Sage.

Berger, A. A. (2012) *Media and Society: A Critical Perspective*. 3rd edn. Rowman and Littlefield Publishers.

Berne, E. (1964) *Games People Play*. USA: Penguin Books.

Bernstein, R. J. (1983) *Beyond Objectivism and Relativism: Science, Hermeneutics and Praxis*. Oxford: Basil Blackwell.

Berry, D. (2007) *Health Communication: Theory and Practice*. Maidenhead, UK: Open University Press.

Bhaskar, R. (1989) *Reclaiming Reality: A Critical Introduction to Contemporary Philosophy*. London: Verso.

Bhaskar, R. (1998) Dialectical critical realism and ethics. In Archer, M., Bhaskar, R., Collier, A., Lawson, T. and Norrie, A. (eds) *Critical Realism. Essential Readings*. London and New York: Routledge, pp. 641–87.

Blaney, C. L. et al. (2012) Validation of the measure of the transtheoretical model for exercise in an adult African-American sample. *American Journal of Health Promotion*, 26 (5), 317–28.

Blue, S., Shove, E., Carmona, C. and Kelly, M. P. (2016) Theories of practice and public health: understanding (un)healthy practices. *Critical Public Health*, 26 (1), 36–50.

Blumler, J. G. and Katz, E. (eds) (1974) *The Uses of Mass Communication*. Newbury Park, CA: Sage.

Bolam, B., Hodgetts, D., Chamberlain, K., Murphy, S. and Gleeson, K. (2003) 'Just do it': an analysis of accounts of control over health amongst lower socioeconomic status groups. *Critical Public Health*, 13, 15–31.

Bonell, C., McKee, M. and Fletcher, A. (2011) Nudge Smudge: UK government misrepresents 'nudge'. *The Lancet*, 377, 2158–9.

Boulos, M. N. K., Gammon, S., Dixon, M. C., MacRury, S. M., Ferusson, M. J., Rodrigues, F. M., Baptista, T. M. and Yang, S. P. (2015) Digital games for Type 1 and Type 2 diabetes: underpinning theory with three illustrative examples. *JMIR Serious Games*, 2015, 3 (1), e3.

Bourdieu, P. and Passeron, J. C. (1990) *Culture Reproduction in Education, Society and Culture*. Trans. from French by R. Nice. London: Sage.

Bourne, A. H. and Robson, M. A. (2009) Perceiving risk and (re)constructing safety: the lived experience of having 'safe' sex. *Health, Risk and Society*, 11, 283–95.

Bowleg, L. (2012) The problem with the phrase women and minorities: intersectionality – an important theoretical framework for public health. *American Journal of Public Health*, 102 (7), 1267–73.

Boyce, T., Robertson, R. and Dixon, A. (2008) *Commissioning and Behaviour Change: Kicking Bad Habits Final Report*. London: The King's Fund.

Boyle, D., Coote, A., Sherwood, C. and Slay, J. (2010) *Right Here, Right Now, Taking Co-Production into the Mainstream*. London: NESTA.

Boyne, R. (2003) *Risk*. Buckingham: Open University Press.

Bradley, I. (2011) Ethical considerations on the use of fear in public health campaigns. *The NYU Langone Online Journal of Medicine*, 23 November 2011. Available at: www.clinicalcorrelations.org/?p=4998

Bradshaw, J. (1972) A taxonomy of social need. In McLachlan, G. (ed.) *Problems and Progress in Medical Care*. Maidenhead: Open University Press.

Branfield, F. and Beresford, P. (2006) *Making User Involvement Work: Supporting Service User Networking and Knowledge*. York: Joseph Rowntree Foundation.

Brannen, J. and Nilsen, A. (2005) Individualisation, choice and structure: a discussion of current trends in sociological analysis. *The Sociological Review*, 53, 412–28.

Breakwell, G. M. (2007) *The Psychology of Risk*. Cambridge: Cambridge University Press.

Brener, N. D., Billy, J. O. G. and Grady, W. R. (2003) Assessment of factors affecting the validity of self-reported health-risk behavior among adolescents: evidence from the scientific literature. *Journal of Adolescent Health*, 33, 436–57.

Brennan, R., Dahl, S. and Eagle, L. (2010) Persuading young consumers to make healthy nutritional decisions. *Journal of Marketing Management*, 26 (7–8), 635–55.

British Institute of Learning Disability (2005) No need to scream: good practice made easy. *Advocacy News*, 20.

Brocklehurst, P. R., Morris, P. and Tickle, M. (2012) Social marketing: an appropriate strategy to reduce oral health inequalities? *International Journal of Health Promotion and Education*, 50 (2), 81–91.

Bronfenbrenner, U. (1974) Developmental research, public policy and the ecology of childhood. *Child Development*, 45 (1), 1–5.

Brookfield, S. D. (1987) *Developing Critical Thinkers: Challenging Adults to Explore Alternative Ways of Thinking and Acting*. San Francisco: Jossey-Bass.

Brown, W. J. and de Matviuk, M. A. C. (2010) Sports celebrities and public health: Diego Maradona's influence on drug use prevention. *Journal of Health Communication*, 15 (4), 358–73.

Buber, M. (1946, 1996) *Paths in Utopia*, 1st edn by Routledge and Kegan Paul, 1st Syracuse University Press edn 1996, New York.

Buber, M. (1958) The I-thou theme, contemporary psychotherapy, and psychodrama. *Pastoral Psychology*, 9 (5), 57–8.

Buber, M. (2004) *Between Man and Man* (1st edn 1947 by Routledge and Kegan Paul, reprinted by Routledge in 1965, 2002 and 2004). London and New York: Routledge.

Buchanan, D. R., Reddy, S. and Hossain, Z. (1994) Social marketing: a critical appraisal. *Health Promotion International*, 9 (1), 49–59.

Bunton, R. (2006) Critical health psychology: Julie Hepworth. *Journal of Health Psychology*, 11, 343–5.

Bunton, R. and Macdonald, G. (2004) *Health Promotion: Disciplines, Diversity and Developments*. 2nd edn. London: Routledge.

Bunton, R., Baldwin, S., Flynn, D. and Whitelaw, S. (2000) The 'stages of change' model in health promotion: science and ideology. *Critical Public Health*, 10, 910, 55–70.

Burke, H. M., Pedersen, K. F. and Williamson, N. E. (2012) An assessment of cost, quality and outcomes for five HIV prevention youth peer education programs in Zambia. *Health Education Research*, 27 (2), 359–69.

Burr, V. (2003) *Social Constructionism*. 2nd edn. London: Routledge.

Butt, J. and O'Neil, A. (2004) *Let's Move On: Black and Minority Ethnic Older People's Views on Research Findings*. York: Joseph Rowntree Foundation.

Campbell, M. A., Finlay, S., Lucas, K., Neal, N. and Williams, R. (2014) Kick the habit: a social marketing campaign by Aboriginal communities in NSW. *Australian Journal of Primary Health*, 20 (4), 327–33.

Cao, Z., Chen, Y. and Wang, S. (2014) Health belief model based evaluation of school health education programme for injury prevention among high school students in the community context. *BMC Public Health*, 14, 26–42.

Carins, J. E. and Rundle-Thiele, S. R. (2013) Eating for the better: a social marketing review (2000–2012). *Public Health Nutrition*, 17 (7), 1628–39.

Carpenter, C. J. (2010) A meta-analysis of the effectiveness of health belief variables in predicting behavior. *Health Communication*, 25 (8), 661–9.

Carrete, L. and Arroyo, P. (2014) Social marketing to improve healthy dietary decisions: insights from a qualitative study in Mexico. *Qualitative Market Research: An International Journal*, 17 (3), 239–63.

Carson, G. (2009) *The Social Model of Disability*. Norwich: The Stationery Office.

Carson, A. J., Chappell, N. L. and Knight, C. J. (2007) Promoting health and innovative health promotion practice through a community arts centre. *Health Promotion Practice*, 8 (4), 366–74.

Carter, T. and Beresford, P. (2000) *Age and Change: Models of Involvement for Older People*. York: Joseph Rowntree Foundation.

Center for Health Strategies Inc. (CHCS) (2000) Fact sheet. *What is Health Literacy?* CHCS, Princeton, NJ, USA. In Kickbusch, I. (2001) Health literacy: addressing the health and education divide. *Health Promotion International*, 16 (3), 289–97.

Central Statistics Office (Ireland): http://www.cso.ie/en/index.html

Centre for Disease Control and Prevention http://www.cdc.gov/healthlit eracy/learn/understandingliteracy.html

Centre for Health Promotion, Women's and Children's Health Network (2012) *Where They Hang Out. Social Media Use in Youth Health Promotion. Analysis Based on a Literature Review and Survey of the Youth Sector in South Australia*. Department of Health, Government of South Australia, Adelaide.

Chalabi, M. (2013) Does a government nudge make us budge? *Guardian*, Tuesday 12 November. Available at www.theguardian.com/politics/2013/ nov/12/government-nudge-theory-budge

Chamberlain, K. (2004) Food and health: expanding the agenda for health psychology. *Journal of Health Psychology*, 9, 467–81.

Chaput, J. P., Klingenberg, L., Astrup, A. and Sjödin, A. M. (2011) Modern sedentary activities promote overconsumption of food in our current obesogenic environment. *Obesity Reviews*, 12 (5), e12–e20.

Christens, B. (2013) In search of powerful empowerment. *Health Education Research*, 28 (3), 371–4.

Chun, J. (2015) Determinants of tobacco use among Korean female adolescents: Longitudinal test of the theory of triadic influence. *Children and Youth Services Review*, 50, 83–7.

Cicero, M. T. (2001) *Cicero on Old Age, on Friendship, on Divination* (trans. by W. A. Falconer). Cambridge, Massachusetts and London, England: Harvard University Press.

Clampitt, P. (2001) *Communicating for Managerial Effectiveness*. 2nd edn. Thousand Oaks, CA: Sage.

Cockerham, W. C. (2005) Health lifestyle theory and the convergence of agency and structure. *Journal of Health and Social Behaviour*, 46, 51–67.

Cohn, S. (2014) From health behaviours to health practices: an introduction. *Sociology of Health and Illness*, 36 (2), 157–62.

Coles, E., Themessl-Huber, M. and Freeman, R. (2012) Investigating community-based health and health promotion for homeless people: a mixed methods review. *Health Education Research*, 27 (4), 624–44.

Connor, M. and Norman, P. (2015) *Predicting and Changing Health Behaviour*. 3rd edn. Maidenhead: Open University Press.

Cook, P. A. and Bellis, M. A. (2001) Knowing the risk: relationships between risk behaviour and health knowledge. *Public Health*, 115, 54–61.

Corbett, M. (2008) The edumometer: The commodification of learning from Galton to the PISA. *Journal for Critical Education Policy Studies*, 6 (1). Available at http://www.jceps.com/archives/576

Corcoran, N. (2011) *Working on Health Communication*. London: Sage.

Corcoran, N. (2013) *Communicating Health: Strategies for Health Promotion*. 2nd edn. London: Sage.

Coulon, S. M. et al. (2012) Formative process evaluation for implementing a social marketing intervention to increase walking among African Americans in the positive action for today's health trial. *American Journal of Public Health*, 102 (12), 2315–23.

Coveney, J. and Bunton, R. (2003) In pursuit of the study of pleasure: implications for health research and practice. *Health*, 7, 161–79.

Crawford, R. (2000) The ritual of health promotion. In Williams, S. J., Gabe, J. and Calnan, M. (eds) *Health, Medicine and Society: Key Theories, Future Agendas*. London and New York: Routledge, pp. 219–35.

Crawford, R. (2006) Health as meaningful social practice. *Health*, 10, 401–20.

Crawshaw, P. (2012) Governing at distance: social marketing and the (bio) politics of responsibility. *Social Science and Medicine*, 75, 200–7.

Crawshaw, P. and Newlove, C. (2011) Men's understanding of social marketing and health: neo-liberalism and health governance. *International Journal of Men's Health*, 10 (2), 136–54.

Cregan, K. (2006) *The Sociology of the Body*. London: Sage.

Crosby, R. A., Salazar, L. F. and DiClemente, R. J. (2013a) Value-expectancy theories. In DiClemente, R. J., Salazar, L. F. and Crosby, R. A. *Health Behaviour Theory for Public Health: Principles, Foundations, and Applications*. Burlington, MA: Jones and Barlett Learning, pp. 65–82.

Crosby, R. A., Salazar, L. F. and DiClemente, R. J. (2013b) Ecological approaches in the new public health. In DiClemente, R. J., Salazar, L. F. and Crosby, R. A. *Health Behaviour Theory for Public Health: Principles, Foundations, and Applications*. Burlington, MA: Jones and Barlett Learning, pp. 231–54.

Cross, R., O'Neil, I. and Dixey, R. (2013) Communicating Health. In Dixey, R. (ed.) *Health Promotion: Global Principles and Practice*. Wallingford: CABI, pp. 78–106.

Crossley, M. L. (2002) 'Could you please pass one of those health leaflets along?': exploring health, morality and resistance through focus groups. *Social Science and Medicine*, 55, 1471–83.

Cruickshank, J. (2012) Positioning positivism, critical realism and social constructionism in the health sciences: a philosophical orientation. *Nursing Inquiry*, 19 (4), 71–82.

Cuban, S. (2006) 'Following the physician's recommendations faithfully and accurately': Functional health literacy, compliance, and the knowledge-based economy. *Journal for Critical Education Policy Studies*, 4 (2). Available at http://www.jceps.com/wp-content/uploads/PDFs/04–2–10.pdf

Culley, S. and Bond, T. (2004) *Integrative Counselling Skills in Action*. 2nd edn. London: Sage.

Daghio, M. M., Fattori, G. and Ciardullo, A. (2006) Evaluation of easy-to-read information material on healthy lifestyles written with the help of citizens' collaboration through networking. *Promotion and Education*, 13 (3), 191–6.

Davies, J. and Macdonald, G. (1998) *Quality, Evidence and Effectiveness in Health Promotion: Striving for Certainties*. London: Routledge.

Davis, S. (2009) *Making an Impact, Adults Learning*. (January) UK: NIACE.

Dempsey, C., Battel-Kirk, B. and Barry, M. M. (2011) *The CompHP core competencies framework for health promotion handbook*. Paris: International Union for Health Promotion and Education.

Denscombe, M. (1993) Personal health and the social psychology of risk-taking. *Health Education Research*, 8, 505–17.

Denscombe, M. (2010) The affect heuristic and perceptions of 'the young smoker' as a risk object. *Health, Risk and Society*, 12, 425–40.

Department for Education and Employment (1999) *A Fresh Start: Improving literacy and numeracy*. The report of the Working Group chaired by Sir Claus Moser. London: DfEE.

Department of Health and Social Security (DHSS) (1980) *Inequalities in Health: Black Report*. London: Penguin Books.

Department of Health (DH) (2001) *The Expert Patient: A New Approach to Chronic Disease Management for the 21st Century*. London: Department of Health.

Department of Health (2002) *Addressing Inequalities – Reaching the Hard-to-Reach Groups*. London: Department of Health.

Department of Health (2007) *Guidance on Joint Strategy Needs Assessment*. Communities and Local Government and Department for Children, Schools and Families. London: Department of Health.

Department of Health (2008a) *Ambitions for Health: A Strategic Framework for Maximising the Potential of Social Marketing and Health-Related Behaviour*. London: Department of Health.

Department of Health (2008b) *Health Inequalities: Progress and Next Steps*. London: Department of Health.

Department of Health (2012) *E-learning for Health Care: e-Learning Programme*. Available at http://www.e-lfh.org.uk/home/

Department of Health (2013a) The Digital Challenge: How a paperless NHS will improve services. Available at http://webarchive.nationalarchives. gov.uk/20150402110949/http://digitalchallenge.dh.gov.uk/2013/01/16/paperless/

Department of Health (2013b) National Mobile Health Worker Project. Final Report. Available at https://www.gov.uk/government/uploads/system/uploads/attachment_data/file/213313/mhwp_final_report.pdf

Dewey, J. (1916) *Democracy and Education*. In Brookfield, S. D. and Preskill, S. (1999) *Discussion as a Way of Teaching – Tools and Techniques for University Teachers*. The Society for Research into Higher Education and Open University Press: London.

Dewey, J. (1933) How we think. A restatement of the relation of reflective thinking to the educative process. In Dewey, J., Boydston, J. A. and Rorty, R., *The Later Works of John Dewey*, vol. 8, 1925–1953.

Dewey, J. (1938, 1997) *Experience and Education*. 1st edn Touchstone. New York: Simon and Schuster.

Dewey, J. (2008) *Democracy and Education*. 2nd edn Cosmo. New Delhi: Cosmo.

DfEE (1999) *A Fresh Start: Improving Literacy and Numeracy*. The Report of the Working Group chaired by Sir Claus Moser. London: Department for Education and Employment.

Dibb, S. and Carrigan, M. (2013) Social marketing transformed: Kotler, Polonsky and Hastings reflect on social marketing in a period of social change. *European Journal of Marketing*, 47 (9), 1376–98.

Dickens, T. E., Johns, S. E. and Chipman, A. (2012) Teenage pregnancy in the United Kingdom: a behavioural ecological perspective. *Journal of Social, Evolutionary, and Cultural Psychology*, 6 (3), 344–59.

DiClemente, R. J., Redding, C. A., Crosby, R. A. and Salazar, L. F. (2013) Stage models for health promotion. In DiClemente, R. J., Salazar, L. F. and Crosby, R. A. *Health Behaviour Theory for Public Health: Principles, Foundations, and Applications*. Burlington, MA: Jones and Barlett Learning, pp. 106–29.

Dickson, D., Saunders, C. and Stringer, M. (1993) *Rewarding People: The Skill of Responding Positively*. London: Routledge.

Dillard, A. J. et al. (2011) The Distinct Role of Comparative Risk Perceptions in a Breast Cancer Prevention Program. *Annals of Behavioral Medicine*, 42, 262–8.

Ding, D. and Gebel, K. (2012) Built environment, physical activity, and obesity: what have we learned from reviewing the literature. *Health Place*, 18: 100–5. Cited in Gubbels, J. S. et al. (2014) The next steps in health behaviour research: the need for ecological modera-tion analyses – an application to diet and physical activity at childcare. *International Journal of Behavioural Nutrition and Physical Activity*, 11 (52) doi:10.1186/1479–5868–11–52.

Dixey, R. (ed.) (2013) *Health Promotion: Global Principles and Practice*. CABI.

Dixey, R., Cross, R. and Foster, S. (2013) The foundations of health promotion. In Dixey, R. (ed.) *Health Promotion: Global Principles and Practice*. Wallingford: CABI, pp. 1–29.

Donovan, R. and Henley, N. (2010) *Principles and Practice of Social Marketing: An International Perspective*. Cambridge: Cambridge University Press.

Dorfman, L. and Krasnow, I. D. (2014) Public health and media advocacy. *Annual Review Public Health*, 35, 293–306.

Dorling, D. (2010) *Injustice, Why Social Inequality Persists*. Bristol, UK and Portland, USA: Policy Press.

Dorling, D. (2015) *Inequality and the 1%*. London and New York: Verso.

Dreibelbis, R. et al. (2013) The integrated behavioural model for water, sanitation, and hygiene: a systematic review of behavioural models and a framework for designing and evaluating behaviour change interventions in infrastructure-restricted settings. *BMC Public Health*, 13, 1015. doi: 10.1186/1471–2458-13-1015.

Dresler-Hawke, E. and Whitehead, D. (2009) The behavioral ecological model as a framework for school-based anti-bullying health promotion interventions. *Journal of School Nursing*, 25 (3), 195–204.

Dutta, M. J. (2008) *Communicating Health: A Culture-Centered Approach*. Cambridge: Polity.

Eakin, J., Robertson, A., Poland, B., Coburn, D. and Edwards, R. (1996) Towards a critical social science perspective on health promotion research. *Health Promotion International*, 11, 157–66.

El-Rahman, A., Mahmoud, A., Amal, M. and Mahmoud, A. (2014) The application of alcohol brief intervention using the health belief model in hospitalised alcohol use disorders patients. *International Journal of Caring Sciences*, 7 (3), 843–56.

Emslie, C. (2005) Women, men and coronary heart disease: a review of the qualitative literature. *Journal of Advanced Nursing*, 51 (4), 382–95.

Evans, D. W. and Hastings, G. (2008) *Public Health Branding: Applying Marketing for Social Change*. Oxford: Oxford University Press.

Evans, D. W. and McCormack, L. (2008) Applying social marketing in health care: communicating evidence to change consumer behaviour. *Medical Decision Making*, 28, 718–31.

Evans, J. (2012) *In Five Years, Most Africans Will Have Smart-Phones*. Available at http://techcrunch.com/2012/06/09/feature-phones-are-not-the-future/

Farr, M., Wardlow, J. and Jones, C. (2008) Tackling health inequalities using geodemographics: a social marketing approach. *International Journal of Market Research*, 50 (4), 449–69.

Field, J. (2006) *Lifelong Learning and the New Educational Order*. 2nd edn. Stoke-on-Trent: Trentham.

Fischer, M. and Lotz, S. (2014) *Is Soft Paternalism Ethically Legitimate? – The*

Relevance of Psychological Processes for the Assessment of Nudge-Based Policies. CGS Working Paper. Vol. 5, no. 2. Germany: University of Cologne. Available at http.//www.cgs.uni-koeln.de/fileadmin/wiso_tak?cgs/pdf/working_paper/cgswp_05_02.pdf

Fjeldsoe, B. S., Marshall, A. L. and Miller, Y. D. (2009) Behaviour change interventions delivered by mobile telephone short-message service. *American Journal of Preventive Medicine*, 36 (2), 165–73. Available at http://www.ncbi.nlm.nih.gov/pubmed/19135907

Flanagan, S. M. and Hancock, B. (2010) 'Reaching the hard to reach': lessons learned from the VCS (voluntary and community sector). A qualitative study. *BMC Health Service Research*, 10 (92). Available at http://www.ncbi.nlm.nih.gov/pmc/articles/PMC2856561/

Flay, B. R. (1999) Understanding environmental, situational and intrapersonal risk and protective factors for youth tobacco use: the Theory of Triadic Influence. *Nicotine and Tobacco Research*, 1, S111–S114.

Fletcher, C. M. (1973) *Communication in Medicine.* Nuffield Provincial Hospital Trust, London. In Bennett, A. E. (1975) *Communication between Doctors and Patients.* Oxford: Oxford University Press.

Flynn, J., Slovic, P. and Kunreuther, H. (eds) (2001) *Risk, Media and Stigma: Understanding Public Challenges to Modern Science and Technology.* London: Earthscan.

Forrest, V., Hunjan, R. and Purtell, R. (2013) *Change in Action: The Ups and Downs of Doing Something Together, Power, Leadership and Identity.* London: PowerHouse.

Foucault, M. (1980) Truth and power. In Gordon, C. (ed.) *Michel Foucault: Power/Knowledge.* London: Harvester Wheatsheaf, pp. 109–33.

Foucault, M. (1997) Sexuality and Solitude. In Rabinow, P. (ed.) *The Essential Works of Michel Foucault. Volume 1: Ethics, Subjectivity, and Truth.* New York: New Press, pp. 298–325.

Fox, N. J. (2012) *The Body.* Cambridge: Polity.

Fox, S. and Jones, S. (2009) *The Social Life of Health Information.* Washington, DC: Pew Internet and American Life Project.

Freire, P. (1972) *Pedagogy of the Oppressed.* Harmondsworth: Penguin.

Freire, P. (1974) Education: domestication or liberation? In Lister, L. (ed.) *Deschooling.* Cambridge: Cambridge University Press.

Freire, P. (1978) *Pedagogy in Progress, the Letters to Guinea Bissau. A Continuum Book.* New York: Seabury Press.

Freire, P. and Freire, A. (2004) *Pedagogy of Hope: Reliving Pedagogy of the Oppressed,* trans. by Robert R. Barr. London, New York: Continuum.

French, J. and Blair-Stevens, C. (2006) *Social Marketing National Benchmark Criteria.* London: UK National Social Marketing Centre. http://www.snh.org.uk/pdfs/sgp/A328466.pdf

French, J., Blair-Stevens, C., McVey, D. and Merritt, R. (eds) (2010) *Social Marketing and Public Health: Theory and Practice.* Oxford: Oxford University Press.

Frerichs, S. (2011) False promises? A sociological critique of the behavioural turn in law and economics. *Journal of Consumer Policy*, 34 (3), 289–314.

Friedman, D. B. and Hoffman-Goertz, L. (2007) An exploratory study of older adults' comprehension of printed cancer information: is readability a key factor? *Journal of Health Communication*, 12 (5), 423–37.

Frohlich, K. L. and Abel, T. (2014) Environmental justice and health practices: understanding how health inequalities arise at the local level. *Sociology of Health and Illness*, 36 (2), 157–62.

Gardner, H. (1983; 1993) *Frames of Mind: The Theory of Multiple Intelligences*. New York: Basic Books.

Gaventa, J. (2006) Finding the spaces for change: a power analysis. In Eyben, R., Harris, C. and Pettit, J. (eds) *Exploring Power for Change*, IDS Bulletin, 37 (6), 23–33.

Gesser-Edelsburg, A., Endevelt, R. and Tirosh-Kamienchick, Y. (2014) Nutrition labelling and the Choices logo in Israel: positioning and perceptions of leading health policy makers. *Journal of Human Nutrition and Dietetics*, 27, 58–68.

Ghahremani, L., Faryabi, R. and Kaveh, M. H. (2013) Effect of health education based on the protection motivation theory on malaria preventative behaviors in rural households of Kerman, Iran. *International Journal of Preventative Medicine*, 5, 463–7.

Gill, R. and Scharff, C. (2011) Introduction. In Gill, R. and Scharff, C. (eds) *New Femininities: Postfeminism, Neoliberalism and Subjectivity*. Basingstoke: Palgrave Macmillan, pp. 1–17.

Gillies, V. and Willig, C. (1997) 'You get the nicotine and that in your blood' – constructions of addiction and control in women's accounts of cigarette smoking. *Journal of Community and Applied Social Psychology*, 7, 285–301.

Giroux, H. A. (1981) *Ideology, Culture and the Process of Schooling*. Philadelphia, London: Temple University Press, Falmer Press.

Gold, J. et al. (2011) A systematic examination of the use of online social networking sites for sexual health promotion. *BioMed Central Public Health*, 11, 583.

Gold, J. et al. (2012) Developing health promotion interventions on social networking sites: recommendations from The Face Space Project. *Journal of Medical Internet Research*, 14 (1), e30. Available at http://www.ncbi.nlm.nih.gov/pmc/articles/PMC3374544/

Golden, S. D. and Earp, J. A. L. (2012) Social ecological approaches to individuals and their contexts: twenty years of health education and behavior health promotion interventions. *Health Education and Behavior*, 39 (3), 364–72.

Goodwin, T. (2012) Why we should reject 'nudge'. *Politics*, 32 (2), 85–92.

Gopaldas, A. (2013) Intersectionality 101. *Journal of Public Policy and Marketing*, 32, 90–4.

Gordon, C. (1980) *Michel Foucault: Power/Knowledge. Selected Interviews and Other Writings 1972–1977.* London: Harvester Wheatsheaf.

Gordon, R. (2013) Unlocking the potential of upstream social marketing. *European Journal of Marketing,* 47 (9), 1525–47.

Gordon, R., McDermott, L., Stead, M. and Angus, K. (2006) The effectiveness of social marketing interventions for health improvement: What's the evidence? *Public Health,* 120, 1133–9.

Graham, D. and Edwards, A. (2013) The psychological burden of obesity: the potential harmful impact of health promotion and education programmes targeting obese individuals. *International Journal of Health Promotion and Education,* 51 (3), 124–33.

Green, A. (2002) The many faces of lifelong learning: recent education policy trends in Europe. *Journal of Education Policy,* 17 (6), 611–26.

Green, J. (2008) Health Education – the case for rehabilitation. *Critical Public Health,* 18 (4), 447–56.

Green, J., Tones, K., Cross, R. and Woodall, J. (2015) *Health Promotion: Planning and Strategies.* 3rd edn. London: Sage.

Grier, S. and Bryant, C. A. (2005) Social marketing in public health. *Annual Review of Public Health,* 26, 319–39.

Griffiths, J., Blair-Stevens, C. and Thorpe, A. (2008) Social marketing for health and specialized health promotion: Stronger together – weaker apart. A paper for debate. London: National Social Marketing Centre and Royal Society for Public Health.

Gubbels, J. S., Van Han, D. H. H., de Vries, N. K., Thijs, C. and Kremers, S. P. J. (2014) The next steps in health behaviour research: the need for ecological moderation analyses – an application to diet and physical activity at childcare. *International Journal of Behavioural Nutrition and Physical Activity,* 11 (52) doi:10.1186/1479–5868–11–52.

Gurrieri, L., Previte, J. and Brace-Goven, J. (2013) Women's bodies as sites of control: inadvertent stigma and exclusion in social marketing. *Journal of Macromarketing,* 33 (2), 128–43.

Hackman, C. L. and Knowlden, A. P. (2014) Theory of reasoned action and theory of planned behaviour-based dietary interventions in adolescents and young adults: a systematic review. *Adolescent Health, Medicine and Therapeutics,* 2014, 5, 101–14.

Hamilton, H. E. and Chou, W. S. (2014) *The Routledge Handbook of Language and Health Communication.* London: Routledge.

Handy, C. (1999) *Inside Organisations.* London: Penguin Books.

Hanson, C., West, J., Beiger, B., Thackeray, R., Barnes, M. and McIntyre, E. (2011) Use and acceptance of social media among health educators. *American Journal of Health Education,* 42 (4), 197–204.

Hargie, O. and Dickson, D. (2004) *Skilled Interpersonal Communication: Research, Theory and Practice.* 4th edn. London: Routledge.

Harris, A. (2005) VII. Discourses of desire as governmentality: young women, sexuality and the significance of safe spaces. *Feminism and Psychology*, 15, 39–43.

Harris, T. A. (2004) *I'm ok – You're ok*. New York: Quill.

Harrison, L., Kelly, P., Lindsay, J., Advocat, J. and Hickey, C. (2011) 'I don't know anyone that has two drinks a day': Young people, alcohol and the government of pleasure. *Health, Risk and Society*, 13, 469–86.

Hart, G. and Carter, S. (2000) A sociology of risk behaviour. In Williams, S. J., Gabe, J. and Calnan, M. (eds) *Health Medicine and Society: Key Theories, Future Agendas*. London: Routledge, pp. 236–54.

Hartley, P. (1999) *Interpersonal Communication*. 2nd edn. London: Routledge.

Hastings, G. and Stead, M. (2006) Social marketing. In Macdowall, W., Bonell, C. and Davies, M. (eds) *Health Promotion Practice*. Maidenhead: Open University Press, pp. 125–38.

Haun, J., Valerio, M., McCormak, L., Sorensen, K. and Paasche-Orlow, M. K. (2014) Health literacy measurement: an inventory and descriptive summary of 51 instruments. *Journal of Health Communication*, (19) 303–33.

Hayden, J. (2014) *Introduction to Health Behaviour Theory*. 2nd edn. Burlington, MA: Jones and Barlett Learning.

Hazelwood, A. (2008) Using text messaging in the treatment of eating disorders. *Nursing Times*, 104 (40), 28–9.

Head, K. J., Noar, S. M., Iannarino, N. T. and Harrington, N. G. (2013) Efficacy of text messaging-based interventions for health promotion: a meta-analysis. *Social Science and Medicine*, 97, 41–8.

Heading, G. (2008) Rural obesity, healthy weight and perceptions of risk: struggles, strategies and motivation for change. *Australian Journal of Rural Health*, 16, 86–91.

Health and Safety Executive (2004) Successful interventions with hard to reach groups. http://www.hse.gov.uk/research/misc/hardtoreach.pdf

Heaney, T. (1996) Adult education for social change: from center stage to the wings and back again. National-Louis University, *ERIC Monograph Online*. Available at http://eric.ed.gov/?id=ED396190

Helèn, I. and Jauho, M. (2003) *Kanslaisuus ja kansanterveys* [Citizenship and Public Health], Helsinki, Gaudeamus. [Abstract]

Hendricks, G., Savahl, S. and Florence, M. (2015) Adolescent peer pressure, leisure boredom, and substance use in low-income Cape Town communities. *Social Behavior and Personality*, 43 (1), 99–110.

Hennink, M., Hutter, I. and Bailey, A. (2011) *Qualitative Research Methods*. London: Sage.

Henwood, F., Wyatt, S., Hart, A. and Smith, J. (2003) 'Ignorance is bliss sometimes': Constraints on the emergences of the 'informed patient' in the changing landscapes of health information. *Sociology of Health and Illness*, 25 (6), 589–607.

Hepworth, J. (2004) The emergence of critical health psychology: can it contribute to promoting public health? *Journal of Health Psychology*, 11, 331–41.

Hoffman, T. and McKenna, K. (2006) Analysis of stroke patients' and carers' reading ability and the content and design of written materials: recommendations for improving written stroke information. *Patient Education and Counselling*, 60 (3), 286–93.

Hoggan, C. (2016) Transformative learning as a metatheory: definition, criteria, and typology. *Adult Education Quarterly*, 66 (1), 57–75.

Horrocks, C. and Johnson, S. (2014) A socially situated approach to inform ways to improve health and wellbeing. *Sociology of Health and Illness*, 36 (2), 175–86.

Horwath, C. C., Schembre, S. M., Motl, R. W., Dishman, R. K. and Nigg, C. R. (2013) Does the transtheoretical model of behavior change provide a useful basis for interventions to promote fruit and vegetable consumption? *American Journal of Health Promotion*, 27 (6), 351–9.

Hoseini, H., Maleki, F., Moeini, M. and Sharifirad, G. R. (2014) Investigating the effect of an education plan based on the health belief model on the physical activity of women who are at risk for hypertension. *Iranian Journal of Nursing and Midwifery Research*, 19 (9), 647–54.

Hou, J. and Shim, M. (2010) The role of provider–patient communication and trust in online sources in internet use for health-related activities. *Journal of Health Communication: International Perspectives*, 15 (s3), 186–99.

Hubley, J. (2004) *Communicating Health: An Action Guide to Health Education and Health Promotion*. 2nd edn. Oxford: Macmillan Education.

Hubley, J. and Copeman, J. with Woodall, J. (2013) *Practical Health Promotion*. 2nd edn. Cambridge: Polity.

Hunjan, R. and Keophilavong, S. (2010) *Power and Making Change Happen*. Dunfermline: Carnegie UK Trust.

Hunjan, R. and Pettit, J. (2011) *Power: A Practical Guide for Facilitating Social Change*. Dunfermline: Carnegie UK Trust.

Illeris, K. (2014) *Transformative Learning and Identity*. London and New York: Routledge.

Institute of Medicine (2002) *Speaking of Health: Assessing Health Communication Strategies for Diverse Populations*. Washington, DC: National Academic Press.

Ioannou, S. (2005) Health logic and health-related behaviours. *Critical Public Health*, 15, 263–73.

Jackson, C. and Tinkler, P. (2007) 'Ladettes' and 'modern girls': 'troublesome' young femininities. *The Sociological Review*, 55, 251–72.

James, K. J., Albrecht, J. A., Litchfield, R. E. and Weishaar, C. A. (2013) A summative evaluation of a food safety social marketing campaign '4-day throw-away' using traditional and social media. *Journal of Food Science Education*, 12, 48–56.

Janssen, M. M., Mathijssen, J. J., van Bon-Martens, M. J., van Oers, H. A. and Garretsen, H. F. (2013) Effectiveness of alcohol prevention interventions based on the principles of social marketing: a systematic review. *Subst Abuse Treat Policy*, 1 (8), doi: 10.1186.1747–597X-8–18.

Jarvis, P. (ed.) (1987) *Twentieth Century Thinkers in Adult Education*. London and New York: Routledge.

Jeffs, T. and Smith, M. K. (1999) *Informal Education. Conversation, Democracy and Learning*. 2nd edn. Ticknall: Education Now Books.

Johnson, R. (1979) 'Really useful knowledge': radical education and working-class culture, 1790–1848. In Clarke, J., Critcher, C. and Johnson, R. (eds) *Working-Class Culture*. New York: St Martin's Press, pp. 75–102.

Jones, A., Bentham, G., Foster, C., Hillsdon, M. and Panter, J. (2007) *Tackling Obesities: Future Choices – Obesogenic Environments. Evidence Review*. London: Department of Innovation, Universities and Skills. Available at www.dius.gov.uk

Joyce, P. (2001) Governmentality and risk: setting priorities in the new NHS. *Sociology of Health and Illness*, 23, 594–614.

Kapetanaki, A. B., Brennan, D. R. and Caraher, M. (2014) Social marketing and healthy eating: findings from young people in Greece. *Int Rev Public Nonprofit Mark*, 11, 161–80.

Kar, S. B. and Alcalay, R. with Alex, S. (eds) (2001a) *Health Communication: A Multicultural Perspective*. London: Sage.

Kar, S. B. and Alcalay, R. with Alex, S. (2001b) Communicating with multicultural populations. In Kar, S. B. and Alcalay, R. with Alex, S. (eds) *Health Communication: A Multicultural Perspective*. London: Sage, pp. 109–37.

Katz, E. and Lazarsfeld, P. (1955) *Personal Influence: The Part Played by People in the Flow of Mass Communication*. Glencoe, IL: Free Press.

Kavas, A. B. (2009) Self-esteem and health-risk behaviours among Turkish late adolescents. *Adolescence*, 44 (173), 187–200.

Kickbusch, I. (2001) Health literacy: addressing the health and education divide. *Health Promotion International*, 16 (3), 289–97.

Kickbusch, I. (2007) Editorial: responding to the health society. *Health Promotion International*, 22, 89–91.

Kickbusch, I. (2009) Health literacy: engaging in a political debate. *International Journal of Public Health*, 131–2.

Kickbusch, I., Pelikan, J. M., Apfel, F. and Tsouros, A. D. (2013) *Health Literacy: The Solid Facts*. Geneva: The Regional Office for Europe, WHO.

Kidd, R. and Kumar, K. (1981) A critical analysis of pseudo-Freirean adult education. *Economic and Political Weekly*, 27–36.

Kiger, A. (2004) *Teaching for Health*. 3rd edn. London: Churchill Livingstone.

King, D., Greaves, F., Exeter, C. and Darzi, A. (2013) 'Gamification': influencing health behaviours with games. *Journal of Royal Society of Medicine*, 106, 76–8.

Kirksey, O., Harper, K., Thompson, S. and Pringle, M. (2004) Assessment of selected patient education materials of various chain pharmacies. *Journal of Health Communication*, 9 (2), 91–3.

Kirsch, I. S. and Jungeblut, A. (1986). *Literacy: Profiles of America's Young Adults*. Princeton, NJ: Educational Testing Service.

Kirsch, I. S., Jungeblut, A. and Campbell, A (1992), *Beyond the School Doors: The Literacy Needs of Job Seekers Served by the US Department of Labor.* ETS Report prepared for the US Department of Labor Employment and Training Administration.

Kirsch, I. S., Jungeblut, A., Jenkins, L. and Kolstad, A. (eds.) (1993), *Adult Literacy in America: A First Look at the Results of the National Adult Literacy Survey.* National Center for Education.

Kirsch, I. S., Jungeblut, A., Jenkins, L. and Kolstad, A. (2002) *National Center For Education Statistics, Adult Literacy in America: A First Look at the Findings of the National Adult Literacy.* US Department of Education, Office of Educational Research and Improvement.

Kirsch, I. and Mosenthal, P. B. (1990). Exploring document literacy: Variables underlying the performance of young adults. *Reading Research Quarterly,* 25(1), 5–30.

Kurlich J. (1992) Adult education through a rear view mirror: the changing face of adult education over the last 25 years. *Convergence* 25(4), 42–7.

Klapper, J. T. (1966) *The Effects of Mass Communication.* London: Free Press.

Knight, P. (2007) *Fostering and Assessing Wicked Competencies.* Available at http://www.open.ac.uk/opencetl/resources/pbpl-resources/knight-2007–fostering-and-assessing-wicked-competencies.

Koch-Weser, S., Bradshaw, Y. S., Gualtieri, L. and Gallagher, S. S. (2010) The internet as a health information source: findings from the 2007 health information national trends survey and implications for health communication. *Journal of Health Communication: International Perspectives,* 15 (s3), 279–93.

Kohut, A., Wilke, R., Menasce, H. J., Simmons, K. and Poushter, J. (2012) Global digital communication: texting, social networking popular worldwide. Available at http://www.pewglobal.org/2011/12/20/global-digital-communication-texting-social-networking-popular-worldwide/

Korp, P. (2008) The symbolic power of 'healthy lifestyles'. *Health Sociology Review,* 1, 18–26.

Koss, V., Azad, S., Gurm, A. and Rosenthal, E. (2012) *This is for Everyone: The Case for Universal Digitisation.* UK: Booz and Company.

Kotler, P., Roberto, N. and Lee, N. (2002) *Social Marketing: Improving the Quality of Life.* 2nd edn. Thousand Oaks, CA: Sage.

Kreuter, M. T. and McClure, S. M. (2004) The role of culture in health communication. *Annual Review Public Health,* 25, 439–55.

Lafferty, N. (2013) *NHS-HE Connectivity Project: Web 2.0 and Social Media in Education and Research.* NHS-HE Connectivity Best Practice Working Group of the NHS-HE Forum.

Lanole, R., Druică, E. and Cornescu, V. (2014) Health knowledge and health consumption in the Romanian society. *Procedia Economics and Finance,* 8, 388–96.

Lasswell, H. D. (1948) The structure and function of communication in society. In McQuail, D. and Windahl, S. (1993) *Communication Models: For the Study of Mass Communication.* 2nd edn. England: Pearson Education Limited.

Last, J. (1987) *Public Health and Human Ecology.* New Jersey: Prentice Hall.

Laverack, G. (2009) *Public Health: Power, Empowerment and Professional Practice.* 2nd edn. London: Palgrave Macmillan.

Laverack, G. (2013) *Health Activism: Foundations and Strategies.* London: Sage.

Lawlor, D. A., Frankey, D. M., Shaw, M., Ebrahim, S., Davey Smith, G. (2003) Smoking and ill health: does lay epidemiology explain the failure of smoking cessation programs among deprived populations? *American Journal of Public Health*, 39, 266–70.

Lawton, R., Connor, M. and McEachen, R. (2009) Desire or reason: predicting health behaviour from affective and cognitive attitudes. *Health Psychology*, 28, 56–65.

Lazarsfeld, P. F. and Merton, R. K. (1955) Mass communication, popular taste and organised social action. In Schramm, W. (ed.) *Mass Communication.* Urbana: University of Illinois Press.

Lazzeri, G. et al. (2014) Factors associated with unhealthy behaviours and health outcomes: a cross-sectional study among Tuscan adolescents (Italy). *International Journal for Equity for Health*, 13, 83–96.

Lee, R. G. and Garvin, T. (2003) Moving from information transfer to information exchange in health and health care. *Social Science and Medicine*, 56, 449–64.

Lefebvre, R. C. (1997) 25 years of social marketing: looking back to the future. *Social Marketing Quarterly* (special issue), 3 (3), 51–8.

Lefebvre, R. C. (2013) *Social Marketing and Social Change: Strategies and Tools for Health, Well-Being, and the Environment.* San Francisco, CA: Jossey-Bass.

Lefebvre, R. C. and Flora, J. A. (1988) Social marketing and public health. *Health Education and Behaviour*, 15 (3), 299–315.

Lemke, T. (2007) An indigestible meal? Foucault, governmentality and state theory. *Scandinavian Journal of Social Theory*, 15, 43–66.

Lenhart, A. (2010) Cell phones and American adults. Pew internet and American life project. Available at http://www.pewinternet.org/2010/09/02/cell-phones-and-american-adults/

Lester, R. T. et al. (2010) Effects of a mobile phone short message service on antiretroviral treatment adherence in Kenya: a randomised trial. *Lancet*, 376, 9755, 1838–45.

Lewin, K. (1948) *Resolving Social Conflicts: Selected Papers on Group Dynamics*, ed. Gertrude Weiss Lewin. New York: Harper and Row.

Lewis, M. A., Mitchell, E. W., Levis, D. M., Isenberg, K. and Kish-Doto, J. (2013) Couples' notions about preconception health: implications for framing social marketing plans. *American Journal of Health Promotion*, 27 (3), no. 3 supplement, 20–9.

Li, Y., Xu, Z. and Liu, S. (2014) Physical activity, self-esteem, and mental health in students from ethnic minorities attending colleges in China. *Social Behavior and Personality*, 42 (4), 529–38.

Lin, P., Simoni, J. M. and Zemon, V. (2005) The health belief model, sexual behaviours and HIV risk among Taiwanese immigrants. *AIDS Education and Research*, 17, 469–83.

Lindridge, A., MacAskill, S., Gnich, W., Eadie, D. and Holme, I. (2013) Applying an ecological model to social marketing communications. *European Journal of Marketing*, 47 (9), 1399–1420.

Lindsay, J. (2010) Health living guidelines and the disconnect with everyday life. *Critical Public Health*, 20, 475–87.

Lister, C., West, J. H., Cannon, B., Sax, T. and Brodegard, D. (2014) Just a fad? Gamification in health and fitness apps. *JMIR Serious Games*, 2 (2), e9.

Local Government Association (2013) *Changing Behaviours in Public Health: To Nudge or to Shove?* London: Local Government Association.

Logie-MacIver, L. and Piacentini, M. G. (2011) Towards a richer understanding of consumer in social marketing contexts: revisiting the stage of change model. *Journal of Marketing Management*, 27 (1–2), 60–76.

Loss, J. and Nagel, E. (2009) Problems and ethical challenges in public health communication. *Bundesgesundheitblatt Gesundheitforschung Gesundheitsschutz*, 52 (5), 502–11 [Abstract only in English].

Loss, J., Lindacher, V. and Curbach, J. (2013) Online social networking sites – a novel setting for health promotion? *Health and Place*, 26, 161–70.

Loss, J., Lindacher, V. and Curbach, J. (2013) Do social networking sites enhance the attractiveness of risky health behaviour? Impression management in adolescents' communication on Facebook and its ethical implications. *Public Health Ethics*, 6. doi: 10.1093/ohe/pht028.

Luca, N. R. and Suggs, L. S. (2012) Theory and model use in social marketing health interventions. *Journal of Health Communication*, 18 (1), 20–40.

Luft, J. and Ingham, H. (1955) *The Johari Window: A Graphic Model for Interpersonal Relations*. University of California at Los Angeles, Extension Office, Western Training Laboratory in Group Development.

Lupton, D. (2003) *Medicine as Culture: Illness, Disease and the Body in Western Societies*. 2nd edn. London: Sage.

Lupton, D. (2006) Sociology and risk. In Mythen, G. and Walklate, S. (eds) *Beyond the Risk Society*. Maidenhead: Open University Press, pp. 11–24.

Lupton, D. (2016) *The Quantified Self*. Cambridge: Polity.

Lynch, M. et al. (2014) Understanding women's preconception health goals: audience segmentation strategies for a preconception health campaign. *Social Marketing Quarterly*, 20, 148–67.

McDermott, L., Stead, M. and Hastings, G. (2005) What is and what is not social marketing: the challenge of reviewing the evidence. *Journal of Marketing Management*, 21, 545–53.

McEachen, R. R. C., Conner, M., Taylor, N. J. and Lawton, R. J. (2011)

Prospective prediction of health-related behaviours with the Theory of Planned Behaviour: A meta-analysis. *Health Psychology Review*, 5 (2), 144–93.

McGuire, W. (1989) Theoretical foundations of campaigns. In Rice, R. and Atkin, C. (eds) *Public Communication Campaigns*. Newbury Park, CA: Sage, pp. 43–65.

McKie, L., Laurier, E., Taylor, R. J. and Lennox, A. S. (2003) Eliciting the smoker's agenda: implications for policy and practice. *Social Science and Medicine*, 56, 83–94.

McLeay, F. J. and Oglethorpe, D. (2013) Social marketing, parental purchasing decisions, and unhealthy food in developing countries: a Nigerian typology. *Journal of Consumer Behaviour*, 12, 232–42.

McQuail, D. (2010) *McQuail's Mass Communication Theory*. 6th edn. London: Sage.

McQuail, D., Blumler, J. G. and Brown, J. (1972) The television audience: a revised perspective. In McQuail, D. (ed.) *Sociology of Mass Communication*. Harmondsworth: Penguin, pp. 135–65.

McQuail, D. and Windahl, S. (1993) *Communication Models: For the Study of Mass Communication*. 2nd edn. England: Pearson Education Limited.

McRobbie, A. (2009) *The Aftermath of Feminism: Gender, Culture and Social Change*. London: Sage.

Machin, S. and Vignoles, A. (2006) *Education Policy in the UK*. Centre for the Economics of Education London School of Economics, Houghton Street, London. Available at http://cee.lse.ac.uk/ceedps/ceedp57.pdf

Mackie, P. (2012) Understanding health literacy. In The evolving concept of health literacy: New directions for health literacy studies. *Journal of Communication in Healthcare*, 8 (1).

Maguire, K. (2006) Health and fear: a study of the use of fear in promoting healthy behaviours among 18–25 year old students in relation to smoking. *Journal of Environmental Health Research*, 5 (2). Available at www.cieh.org/jehr/health_and_fear_a_study.html

Maibach, E. and Parrott, R. (1995) *Designing Health Messages: Approaches from Communication Theory and Public Health Practice*. London: Sage.

Manning, M. (2009) The effects of subjective norms on behaviour in the theory of planned behaviour: a meta-analysis. *British Journal of Social Psychology*, 48, 649–705.

Mantoura, P. and Potvin, L. (2012) A realist-constructionist perspective on participatory research in health promotion. *Health Promotion International*, 28 (1), 61–72.

Manyozo, L. (2012) Community media, health communication, and engagement: a theoretical matrix. In Obregon, R. and Waisbord, S. (eds) *The Handbook of Global Health Communication*. Chichester: Wiley-Blackwell.

Marmot, M. (2006) Harveian oration: health in an unequal world. *The Lancet*, 368, 2081–94.

Marmot, M. (2010) *Fair Society Healthy Lives: The Marmot Review.* The Marmot Review. Strategy Review of Health Inequality post 2010.

Marshall, S. (2012) Health literacy in Ireland: reading between the lines. The evolving concept of health literacy: new directions for health literacy studies. *Journal of Communication in Healthcare,* 8 (1).

Marshall, S. J. and Biddle, S. J. H. (2001) The transtheoretical model of behaviour change: a meta-analysis of applications to physical activity and exercise. *Ann. Behav. Med,* 23 (4), 229–46.

Martin, B. (1988) Feminism, criticism and Foucault. In Diamond, I. and Quinby, F. (eds) *Feminism and Foucault: Reflections and Resistance.* Boston: North-Eastern University Press, pp. 3–22.

Martin, S. et al. (2011) Effectiveness and impact of networked communication interventions in young people with mental health conditions: a systematic review. *Patient Education and Counselling,* 85, e108–e119.

Martínez Donate, A. P. et al. (2010) *Hombres sanos:* evaluation of a social marketing campaign for heterosexually identified Latino men who have sex with men and women. *American Journal of Public Health,* 100, 2532–40.

Maslow, A. H. (1970) *Motivation and Personality.* 2nd edn. New York: Harper and Row.

Mason-Jones, A. J., Flisher, A. J. and Mathews, C. (2011) Who are the peer educators? HIV prevention in South African schools. *Health Education Research,* 26 (3), 563–71.

Mauger, S., Deuchars, G., Sexton, S. and Schehrer, S. (2010) *Involving Users in Commissioning Local Services.* York: Joseph Rowntree Foundation.

Mayo, M. and Thompson, J. (1995) *Adult Learning, Critical Intelligence and Social Change.* Leicester: National Institute of Adult Continuing Education.

Measham, F. and Brain, K. (2005) 'Binge' drinking, British alcohol policy and the new culture of intoxication. *Crime Media Culture,* 1, 262–83.

Measham, F. and Shiner, M. (2009) The legacy of 'normalisation': the role of classical and contemporary criminological theory in understanding young people's drug use. *International Journal of Drug Policy,* 20, 502–8.

Ménard, J. (2010) A 'nudge' for public health ethics: libertarian paternalism as a framework for ethical analysis of public health interventions. *Public Health Ethics,* 3 (3), 229–38.

Mendelovits, J. (2011) *IALS (International Adult Literacy Survey): Its Meaning and Impact for Policy and Practice.* October 23–25, Banff, Alberta.

Mendelsohn, H. (1968) Which shall it be: mass education or mass persuasion for health? *American Journal for Public Health,* 58, 131–7.

Mezirow, J. (1997) *Transformative Learning: Theory to Practice. New Directions for Adult and Continuing Education. No. 74.* San Francisco: Jossey-Bass Publishers.

Michie, S., Hyder, N., Walia, A. and West, R. (2010) Development of a taxonomy of behaviour change techniques used in individual behavioural support for smoking cessation. *Addictive Behaviors,* 36 (4), 315–19.

Michie, S., van Stralen, M. M. and West, R. (2011) The behaviour change wheel: A new method for characterising and designing behaviour change interventions. *Implementation Science*, 6, 42–53.

Mielewczyk, F. and Willig, C. (2007) Old clothes and an older look: the case for a radical makeover in health behaviour research. *Theory and Psychology*, 17, 811–37.

Milana, M. and Nesbit, T. (eds) (2015) *Global Perspectives on Adult Education and Learning Policy*. London: Palgrave Macmillan.

Miller, A. S., Cafazzo, J. A. and Seto, E. (2014) A game plan: gamification design principles in health applications for chronic disease management. *Health Informatics Journal*, 22, 184–93.

Miller, P. G. (2005) Scapegoating, self-confidence and risk-comparison: the functionality of risk neutralizations and lay epidemiology by injecting drug users. *The International Journal of Drug Policy*, 16, 246–53.

Miniwatts Marketing Group (2012) *Internet Usage Statistics*. The Internet Big Picture. World Internet Users and Population Stats.

Mitchell, W. A., Crawshaw, P., Bunton, R. and Green, E. E. (2001) Situating young people's experiences of risk and identity. *Health, Risk and Society*, 3, 217–33.

Moore, D. (2008) Erasing pleasure from public discourse on illicit drugs: on the creation and reproduction of an absence. *International Journal of Drug Policy*, 19, 353–8.

Moore, S. E. H. (2010) Is the healthy body gendered? Toward a feminist critique of the new paradigm of health. *Body and Society*, 16, 95–118.

Morgan, A. and Ziglio, E. (2007) Revitalising the evidence base for public health: an assets model. *International Union for Health Promotion and Education – Promotion and Education Supplement*, 14, 17–22.

Murray, T. S., Kirsch, I. S., and Jenkins, L. (eds.) (1997) *Adult Literacy in OECD Countries: Technical Report on the First International Adult Literacy Survey*. National Center for Education Statistics, United States Department of Education, Washington, DC.

Murtha, M. (2015) Health literacy can increase compliance. *ASBN Update*, 19 (2), 10–11.

National Research and Development Centre (NRDC) (2011) *Work, Society and Lifelong Literacy: Report of the Inquiry into Adult Literacy in England*. London: Institute of Education.

National Social Marketing Centre (2007, 2010) www.thensmc.cpm

Nery Suárez Lugo, C. (2013) Social marketing as a supporting tool for sexual health in Cuba. *Revista Cubana de Salud Pública*, 39 (5), 950–60.

Nettleton, S. (2006) *The Sociology of Health and Illness*. 2nd edn. Cambridge: Polity.

Nettleton, S. and Green, J. (2014) Thinking about changing mobility practices: how a social practice approach can help. *Sociology of Health and Illness*, 36 (2), 157–62.

Newton, J. D., Newton, F. J., Turk, T. and Ewing, M. (2013) Ethical evaluation of audience segmentation social marketing. *European Journal of Marketing*, 47 (9), 1421–38.

NHS Five Year Forward View (2014) Available at http://www.england.nhs. uk/ourwork/futurenhs/

NHS Patient Information (2008) Available at http://www.institute.nhs.uk/ quality_and_service_improvement_tools/quality_and_service_improve ment_tools/patient_information.html

Noar, S. M. (2008) Behavioural interventions to reduce HIV-related sexual risk behaviour: review and synthesis of meta-analytic evidence. *AIDS and Behaviour*, 12 (3), 335–53.

Norman, C. and Skinner, H. (2006) eHealth literacy: essential skills for consumer health in a networked world. *J Med Internet Res.* 8 (2), doi: 10.2196/ jmir.8.2.e9

Nuffield Council on Bioethics (2007) *Public Health Ethical Issues*. London: Nuffield Council on Bioethics.

Nutbeam, D. (1998) The challenge to provide 'evidence' in health promotion. *Health Promotion International*, 14 (2), 99–101.

Nutbeam, D. (2000) Health literacy as a public health goal: a challenge for contemporary health education and communication strategies into the 21st century. *Health Promotion International*, 15 (3), 259–67.

Nutbeam, D. (2008) The evolving concept of health literacy. *Social Science and Medicine*, 67 (12), 2072–8.

O'Hara, L., Taylor, J. and Barnes, M. (2015) We are all ballooning: multimedia critical discourse analysis of *measure up* and *swap it, don't stop it* social marketing campaigns. *Media-Culture Journal*, 18 (3), 1–11.

Oliver, A. (2013) From nudging to budging: using behavourial economic to inform public sector policy. *Journal of Social Policy*, doi:10.1017/ S0047279413000299

Ong, B. N. et al. (2014) Behaviour change and social blinkers? The role of sociology in trials of self-management behaviour in chronic conditions. *Sociology of Health and Illness*, 36 (2), 226–38.

ONS Online National Statistics: https://www.ons.gov.uk

Organization for Economic Co-operation and Development (1992) *Adult Illiteracy and Economic Performance*. Paris, France: Author

Organization for Economic Co-operation and Development / Organisation de Coopération et de Développement Economiques, and Human Resources Development Canada (1997) *Literacy Skill for the Knowledge Society: Further Results of the International Adult Literacy Survey*. Paris and Ottawa: OECD.

Organization for Economic Co-operation and Development, Paris, and the Minister of Industry, Canada (2000) *Literacy in the Information Age, Final Report of the International Adult Literacy Survey*. OECD.

O'Rourke, R. (1995) All equal now? In Mayo, M. and Thompson, J. (eds) *Adult Learning, Critical Intelligence and Social Change*. Leicester: National Institute of Adult Continuing Education.

Parker, G. (1990) *With Due Care and Attention: A Review of Research on Informal Care.* 2nd edn. London: Family Policy Studies Centre.

Parker, J. and Stanworth, H. (2005) 'Go for it!' Towards a critical realist approach to voluntary risk-taking. *Health, Risk and Society,* 7, 319–36.

Parker, R. M. and Guzmararian, J. A. (2003) Health literacy: essential for health communication. *Journal of Health Communication,* 8 (s1), 116–18.

Patel, M. S., Asch, D. A., Volpp, K. G. (2015) Wearable devices as facilitators, not drivers, of health behavior change. *JAMA,* 313 (5), 459–60.

Patton, M. Q. (2002) *Qualitative Research and Evaluation Methods.* 3rd edn. London: Sage.

Pawlyn, J. (2012) The use of e-learning in continuing professional development. *Learning Disability Practice,* 15 (1), 33–7.

Peerson, A. and Saunders, M. (2009) Health literacy revisited: what do we mean and why does it matter? *Health Promotion International,* 24 (3), 285–96.

Peters, J. M. and Bell, B. (1987) Horton of Highlander. In Jarvis, P. (ed.) *Twentieth Century Thinkers in Adult Education.* London and New York: Routledge.

Peterson, A., Davis, M., Fraser, S. and Lindsay, J. (2010) Healthy living and citizenship: an overview. *Critical Public Health,* 20, 391–400.

Peterson, A. and Lupton, D. (1996) *The New Public Health: Health and Self in the Age of Risk.* St Leonards, Australia: Allen and Unwin.

Pfeiffer, J. (2004) Condom social marketing, pentecostalism, and structural adjustment in Mozambique: a clash of AIDS prevention messages. *Medical Anthropology Quarterly,* 18 (11), 77–103.

Phipps, A. (2014) *The Politics of the Body.* Cambridge: Polity.

Pickett, K. and Wilkinson, R. (2009) *The Spirit Level: Why Equality is Better for Everyone.* London: Penguin.

Pidgeon, N., Henwood, K. and Macguire, B. (2001) Public health communication and the social amplification of risks: present knowledge and future prospects. In Bennett, P. and Calman, K. (eds) *Risk Communication and Public Health.* Oxford: Oxford University Press, pp. 64–77.

Pilkington, H. (2007) In good company: risk, security and choice in young people's drug decisions. *The Sociological Review,* 55, 373–92.

Pleasant, A. and Kuruvilla, S. (2008) A tale of two health literacies: public health and clinical approaches to health literacy. *Health Promotion International,* 23, 152–9.

Pleasant, A., McKinney, J. and Rikard, R. V. (2011) Health literacy measurement: a proposed research agenda. *Journal of Health Communication,* 16, 11–21.

Plotnikoff, R. C., Costigan, S. A., Karunamuni, N. and Lubans, D. R. (2013) Social cognitive theories used to explain physical activity behaviour in adolescents: a systematic review and meta-analysis. *Preventive Medicine,* 56, 245–53.

Polanyi, M., McIntosh, T. and Kosny, A. (2005) Understanding and improving the health of workers in the new economy: a call for a participatory dialogue-based approach to work-health related research. *Critical Public Health*, 15 (2), 103–19.

Polič, M. (2009) Decision making, between rationality and reality. *Interdisciplinary Description of Complex Systems*, 7, 78–89.

Popay, J., Williams, G., Thomas, C. and Gatrell, T. (1998) Theorising inequalities in health: the place of lay knowledge. *Sociology of Health and Illness*, 20, 619–44.

Portnoy, D. B., Ferrer, R. A., Bergman, H. E., Klein, W. M. P. (2014) Changing deliberative and affective responses to health risk: a meta-analysis. *Health Psychology Review*, 8 (3), 296–318.

Potter, J. (1998) Fragments in the realization of relativism. In Parker, I. (ed.) *Social constructionism, discourse and realism*. London: Sage, pp. 27–45.

Potter, J. (2003) *Representing Reality: Discourse, Rhetoric and Social Constructionism*. London: Sage.

Prata, N., Weidert, K., Fraser, A. and Gessessew, A. (2011) Meeting rural demand: a case for combining community-based distribution and social marketing of injectable contraceptives in Tigray, Ethiopia. *PLOS One*, doi: 10.1371/journal.pone.0068794

Pratt, D. D. and Associates (2005) *Five Perspectives on Teaching in Adult and Higher Education – Reprint of the 1998 Edition with Corrections*. Florida: Krieger Publishing Company.

Prestwich, A. et al. (2013) Does theory influence the effectiveness of health behavior interventions? Meta-analysis. *Health Psychology*, 33 (5), 465–74.

Prior, L. (2003) Belief, knowledge and expertise: the emergence of the lay expert in medical sociology. *Sociology of Health and Illness*, 25, 41–57.

Prochaska, J. O. and DiClemente, C. C. (1984) *The Transtheoretical Approach: Towards a Systematic Eclectic Framework*. Homeward, IL: Dow Jones Irwin.

Public Health England (2015) *Review of the Public Health Skills and Knowledge Framework (PHSKF): Report on a Series of Consultations*, Spring 2015. London: Public Health England.

Qureshi, N. and Shaikh, B. T. (2006) Myths, fallacies and misconceptions: applying social marketing for promoting appropriate health seeking behavior in Pakistan. *Anthropology and Medicine*, 13 (2), 131–9.

Rai-Atkins, A. et al. (2002) *Best Practice in Mental Health*. Bristol: Policy Press.

Raphael, D. (2000) The question of evidence in health promotion. *Health Promotion International*, 15 (4), 355–67.

Raphael, D. (2008) Beyond positivism: public scholarship in support of health. *Antipode*, 40 (3), 404–13.

Ratzan, S. C. (2011a) Connecting the MDGs and NCDs with digital health. *Journal of Health Communication: International Perspectives*, 16 (7), 681–5.

Ratzan, S. C. (2011b) Health information: diffusing information to knowledge and action. *Journal of Health Communication: International Perspectives*, 16 (9), 923–4.

Ratzan, S. C. (2011c) Our new 'social' communication age in health. *Journal of Health Communication: International Perspectives*, 16 (8), 803–4.

Rhodes, J., Spencer, R., Saito, R. and Sipe, C. (2006) Online mentoring: the promise and challenges of an emerging approach to youth development. *Journal of Primary Prevention*, 27 (5), 497–513.

Rhodes, R. E. and de Bruijn, G. (2013) How big is the physical activity intention-behaviour gap? A meta-analysis using the action control framework. *British Journal of Health Psychology*, 18, 296–309.

Rhodes, R. E. and Dickau, L. (2012) Experimental evidence for the intention-behavior relationship in the physical activity domain: a meta-analysis. *Health Psychology*, 31 (6), 724–7.

Rice, R. E. and Atkin, C. K. (2009) Public communication campaigns: theoretical principles and practical applications. In Bryant, J. and Oliver, M. (eds) *Media Effects: Advances in Theory and Research*. 3rd edn. Hillsdale, NJ: Lawrence Erlbaum Associates, pp. 436–68.

Rich, E. and Evans, J. (2008) Learning to be healthy, dying to be thin: the representation of weight via body perfection codes in schools. In Riley, S., Burns, M., Frith, H., Wiggins, S. and Markula, P. (eds) *Representations, Identities and Practices of Weight and Body Management*. Basingstoke: Palgrave Macmillan, pp. 60–76.

Rimal, R. N. and Lakinski, M. K. (2009) Why health communication is important to public health. *Bulletin of the World Health Organization*, 87, 247–8.

Robertson, S. (2006) 'Not living life in too much of an excess': lay men understanding health and well-being. *Health*, 10, 175–89.

Robertson, S. and Williams, R. (2010) Men, public health and health promotion: towards a critically structural and embodied understanding. In Gough, B. and Robertson, S. (eds) *Men, Masculinities and Health: Critical Perspectives*. Basingstoke: Palgrave Macmillan, pp. 48–66.

Robinson, M. and Robertson, S. (2010) The application of social marketing to promoting men's health: a brief critique. *International Journal of Men's Health*, 9 (1), 50–61.

Rochlen, A. B. and Hoyer, W. D. (2005) Marketing mental health to men: theoretical and practical considerations. *Journal of Clinical Psychology*, 61 (6), 675–84.

Rodham, K. (2010) *Health Psychology*. Basingstoke: Palgrave Macmillan.

Rogers, C. R. (1961) *On Becoming a Person. A Therapist's View of Psychotherapy*. Boston: Houghton Mifflin.

Rogers, C. R. (1969) *Freedom to Learn*. New York: Merrill.

Rogers, C. R. (1980) *A Way of Being*. Boston: Houghton Mifflin.

Rogers, E. M. (1986) *Communication Technology: The New Media in Society*. New York: The Free Press.

Rogers, E. M. (1995) *The Diffusion of Innovations*. 4th edn. New York: The Free Press.

Rogers, E. M. (2003) *Diffusion of Innovations*. 5th edn. New York: The Free Press.

Rogers, E. M. and Shocmakei, F. (1971) *The Communication of Innovations*. New York: The Free Press.

Rogers, R. W. (1975) A protection motivation theory of fear appeals and attitude change. *Journal of Psychology*, 91, 93–114.

Rogers, R. W. (1983) Cognitive and physiological processes in fear appeals and attitude change: a revised theory of protection motivation. In Cacippo, J. R. and Petty, R. E. (eds) *Social Psychology: A Source Book*. New York: Guilford Press, pp. 153–76.

Room, R. (2011) Addiction and personal responsibility as solutions to the contradictions of neoliberal consumerism. *Critical Public Health*, 21, 141–51.

Rose, N. (2000) Risk, trust and scepticism in the age of the new genetics. In Adam, B., Beck, U. and Van Loon, J. (eds) *The Risk Society and Beyond: Critical Issues for Social Theory*. London: Sage, pp. 63–77.

Rose, N. and Miller, P. (2010) Political power beyond the state: problematics of government. *The British Journal of Sociology*, 271–303.

Rose, N., O'Malley, P. and Valverde, M. (2006) Governmentality. *Annual Review of Law and Social Science*, 2, 83–104.

Rowlands, G. (2012) Health literacy and public health: a framework for developing skills and empowering citizens. *Perspectives in Public Health*, 132 (1).

Roy, S. C. (2008) 'Taking charge of your health': discourses of responsibility in English-Canadian women's magazines. *Sociology of Health and Illness*, 30, 463–77.

Rudatsikira, E., Muula, A. S., Mulenga, D. and Siziya, S. (2012) Prevalence and correlates of obesity among Lusaka residents, Zambia: a population-based survey. *International Archives of Medicine*, 5 (14), doi: 10.1186/1755–7682–5–14

Rudd, R. E. (2010) The health literacy environment activity packet: *First Impressions and A Walking Interview*.

Rudd, R. E. (2012) Oral health literacy: correcting the mismatch. *Journal of Public Health Dentistry*, 72 (s31), doi: 10.1111/j.1752–7325. 2011.00299

Rudd, R. E. (2015) The evolving concept of health literacy: new directions for health literacy studies. *Journal of Communication in Healthcare*, 8 (1).

Saghai, Y. (2013) Salvaging the concept of nudge. *Journal of Medical Ethics*, 39, 487–93.

Salazar, L. F., Crosby, R. A., Noar, S. M., Walker, J. H. and DiClemente, R. J. (2013) Models based on perceived threat and fear appeals. In DiClemente, R. J., Salazar, L. F. and Crosby, R. A. *Health Behaviour Theory for Public Health: Principles, Foundations, and Applications*. Burlington, MA: Jones and Barlett Learning, pp. 83–104.

Sanders, T. (2006) Sexuality and risk. In Mythen, G. and Walklate, S. (eds)

Beyond the Risk Society: Critical Reflections on Risk and Human Security.
Maidenhead: Open University Press, pp. 96–113.

Sarafino, E. P. and Smith, T. W. (2011) *Health Psychology: Biopsychosocial Interactions.* 7th edn. New Jersey: John Wiley and Sons.

Sargant, N. and Aldridge, F. (2002) *Adult Learning and Social Division: A Persistent Pattern. Vol. 1.* Leicester: NIACE.

Sargant, N. et al. (1997) *The Learning Divide.* Leicester: NIACE.

Scanfeld, D., Scanfeld, V. and Larson, E. L. (2010) Dissemination of health information through social networks: Twitter and antibiotics. *American Journal of Infection Control,* 38 (3), 182–8.

Schellenberg, J. R. A. et al. (2001) Effect of large-scale social marketing of insecticide-treated nets on child survival in rural Tanzania. *Lancet,* 357, 1241–7.

Schnellenbach, J. R. A. (2012) Nudges and norms: on the political economy of soft paternalism. *European Journal of Political Economy,* 28 (2), 266–77.

Schramm, W. (1954) How communication works. In Schramm, W. (ed.) *The Process and Effects of Mass Communication.* Urbana: University of Illinois Press. In McQuail, D. and Windahl, S. (1993) *Communication Models: For the Study of Mass Communication.* 2nd edn. England: Pearson Education Limited.

Schwartz, B. (2004) *The Paradox of Choice: Why More is Less.* London: Harper Perennial.

Science and Technology Select Committee (2011) *Behaviour Change. 2nd Report of Session 2010–12.* London: The Stationery Office.

Sears, A. (2003) *Retooling the Mind Factory: Education in a Lean State.* Aurora (ONT): Garamond Press.

Shannon, C. and Weaver, W. (1949) The mathematical theory of communication. Urbana: University of Illinois Press. In McQuail, D. and Windahl, S. (1993) *Communication Models: For the Study of Mass Communication.* 2nd edn. England: Pearson Education Limited.

Shariful Islam, S. M. and Tabassum, R. (2015) Implementation of information and communication technologies for health in Bangladesh. *Bulletin of the World Health Organization,* 93, 806–9.

Sharpe, R., Beetham, H. and De Freitas, S. (2010) *Rethinking Learning for a Digital Age – How Learners are Shaping their Own Experiences.* London: Routledge.

Shaw, M. and Crowther, J. (1995) Beyond supervision. In Mayo, M. and Thompson, J. (eds) *Adult Learning, Critical Intelligence and Social Change.* Leicester: National Institute of Adult Continuing Education.

Shiller, R. J., Nobel Prize Winner: 'Inequality biggest problem facing US', *Digital Journal,* 15 October 2013. Available at digitaljournal.com.

Shilling, C. (1993) *The Body and Social Theory.* London: Sage.

Shoveller, J. A. and Johnson, J. L. (2006) Risky groups, risky behaviour, and risky persons: dominating discourses on youth sexual health. *Critical Public Health,* 16, 47–60.

Siemens, G. (2005) *Connectivism: Learning as Network Creation*. Available at http://www.elearnspace.org/Articles/networks.htm

Silva, P., Lott, R., Mota, J. and Welk, G. (2014) Direct and indirect effects of social support on youth physical activity behaviour. *Pediatric Exercise Science*, 26, 86–94.

Sindall, C. (2002) Does health promotion need a code of ethics? *Health Promotion International*, 17 (3), 201–3.

Sinden, D. and Wister, A. V. (2008) E-health promotion for aging baby boomers in North America. *Gerontechnology*, 7 (3), 271–8.

Sixsmith, J., Doyle, P., D'Eath, M. and Barry, M. M. (2014) *Health Communication and its Role in the Prevention and Control of Communicable Disease in Europe: Current Evidence, Practice and Future Developments*. Stockholm: ECDC.

Smith, C. (2002) Punishment and pleasure: women, food and the imprisoned body. *Sociological Review*, 197–214.

Smith, D. (2014) Internet use on mobile phones in Africa predicted to increase 20-fold. *Guardian Online*. Available at http://www.theguardian.com/world/2014/jun/05/internet-use-mobile-phones-africa-predicted-increase-20–fold

Smith, M. (1994) *Local Education: Community, Conversation and Praxis*. Buckingham, UK: Open University Press.

Smith, M. K. (1999, 2011) 'What is praxis?' in the encyclopaedia of informal education. Available at http://www.infed.org/biblio/b-praxis.htm

Sniehotta, F. F., Presseau, J. and Araújo-Soares, V. (2014) Time to retire the theory of planned behaviour. *Health Psychology Review*, 8 (1), 1–7.

Snyder, F. and Flay, B. R. (2012) Brief introduction to the theory of triadic influence. Unpublished document. Oregon State University. August 2012. Available at https://people.oregonstate.edu

Sood, S., Shefner-Rogers, C. and Skinner, J. (2014) Health communication campaigns in developing countries. *Journal of Creative Communications*, 9 (1), 67–84.

Soto Mas, F. G., Kane, W. M., Ford, E. S., Marshall, J. R., Staten, L. K. and Smith, J. E. (2000) *Camine con Nosotros*: connecting theory and practice for promoting physical activity among hispanic women. *Health Promotion Practice*, 1 (2), 178–87.

South, J., White, J. and Gamsu, M. (2013) *People Centred Public Health*. Bristol: Policy Press.

Springett, J., Owens, C. and Callaghan, J. (2007) The challenge of combining 'lay' knowledge with 'evidence-based' practice in health promotion: fag ends smoking cessation service. *Critical Public Health*, 17 (3), 243–56.

Stainton-Rogers, W. (2011) *Social Psychology*. 2nd edn. Maidenhead: Open University Press.

Stainton-Rogers, W. (2012) Changing behaviour: can critical psychology influence policy and practice? In Horrocks, C. and Johnson, S. (eds)

Advances in Health Psychology: Critical Approaches. Basingstoke: Palgrave Macmillan, pp. 44–59.

Statistics Canada (1991) *Adult Literacy in Canada: Results of a National Study.* Ottawa, Statistics Canada Catalogue no. 89-525-XPE. 101 p.

Statistics Canada (2000, 2005) *International Adult Literacy Survey, Microdata User's Guide.* Published by Web Culture, Tourism and the Centre for Education Statistics. Available at www.statcan

Stead, M. and Gordon, R. (2010) Providing evidence for social marketing's effectiveness. In French, J., Blair-Stevens, D. and Merritt, R. (eds) *Social Marketing and Public Health: Theory and Practice.* Oxford: Oxford University Press, pp. 81–96.

Stephens, C. (2008) *Health Promotion: A Psychosocial Approach.* Maidenhead: Open University Press.

Stevenson, F. A., Kerr, C., Murray, E. and Nazareth, I. (2007) Information from the Internet and the doctor-patient relationship: The patient perspective – a qualitative study. *BMC Family Practice*, 8, 47.

Stuart, A. and Donaghue, N. (2012) Choosing to conform: the discursive complexities of choice in relation to feminine beauty practices. *Feminism and Psychology*, 22, 98–121.

Svenson, G., Burke, H. and Johnson, L. (2008) *Impact of Youth Peer Education Programs: Final Results from an FHI/YouthNet Study in Zambia.* Youth Research Working Paper No. 9. NC, USA: Family Health International.

Swami, V. et al. (2009) Lay perceptions of current and future health, the causes of illness, and the nature of recovery: explaining health and illness in Malaysia. *British Journal of Health Psychology*, 14, 519–40.

Sweeney, A. M. and Moyer, A. (2015) Self-affirmation and responses to health messages: a meta-analysis on intentions and behavior. *Health Psychology*, 34 (2), 149–59.

Sychareun, V. et al. (2013) Predictors of premarital sexual activity among unmarried youth in Vientiane, Lao PDR: The role of parent-youth interaction and peer influence. *Global Public Health*, 8 (8), 958–75.

Sykes, S., Willis, J., Rowlands, G. and Popple, K. (2013) Understanding Critical health literacy: a concept analysis, *BMC Public Health*, DOI: 10.1186/1471-2458-13-150.

Sylvester, O. A. (2014) Influence of self-esteem, parenting style and parental monitoring on sexual risk behaviour of adolescents in Ibadan. *Gender and Behaviour*, 12 (2), 6341–53.

Tannahill, A. (2008) DEBATE. Beyond evidence to ethics: a decision-making framework for health promotion, public health and health improvement. *Health Promotion International*, 23 (4), 380–90.

Taylor, P. (1993) *The Texts of Paulo Freire.* Buckingham: Open University Press.

Taylor, P. (2007) The lay contribution to public health. In Orme, J., Powell, J., Taylor, P. and Grey, M. *Public Health in the 21st Century: New*

Perspectives on Policy, Participation and Practice. 2nd edn. Buckingham: Open University Press.

Taylor, M., Dlamini, N., Khanyile, Z., Mpanza, L. and Sathiparsad, R. (2012) Exploring the use of role play in a school-based programme to reduce teenage pregnancy. *South African Journal of Education,* 32 (4), 441–8.

Tengland, P. (2012) Behaviour change or empowerment: on the ethics of health promotion strategies. *Public Health Ethics,* 5, 140–53.

Thaler, C. R. and Sunstein, R. H. (2008) *Nudge: Improving Decisions about Health, Health and Happiness.* Boston, NE: Yale University Press.

Thompson, J. (1993) Learning, liberation and maturity. An open letter to whoever's left. *Adults Learning,* 4 (9), 244.

Thompson, L. and Kumar, A. (2011) Responses to health promotion campaigns: resistance, denial and othering. *Critical Public Health,* 21, 105–17.

Thrasher, J. F., Huang, L., Pérez-Hernández, R., Neiderdeppe, J., Arillo-Santillán, E. and Alday, J. (2011) Evaluation of a social marketing campaign to support Mexico City's comprehensive smoke-free law. *American Journal of Public Health,* 101 (2), 328–35.

Tones, K. (1999) Evaluating health promotion: a tale of three errors. *Patient Education and Counselling,* 39, 227–36.

Tones, K. (2002) Health literacy: new wine in old bottles? *Health Education Research,* 17 (3), 287–90.

Tulloch, J. and Lupton, D. (2003) *Risk and Everyday Life.* London: Sage.

Turner, M. M. (2012) Using emotional appeals in health messages. In Cho, H. (2012) *Health Communication Message Design: Theory and Practice.* London: Sage.

Tyson, M., Covey, J. and Rosenthal, H. E. S. (2014) Theory of planned behavior interventions for reducing heterosexual risk behaviors: a meta-analysis. *Health Psychology,* 33 (12), 1454–67.

UNAIDS (1999) *Peer Education and HIV/AIDS: Concepts, Uses and Challenges: Report of a Consultation.* Geneva, Switzerland: Joint United Nations Programme on HIV/AIDS (UNAIDS).

Upton, D. and Thirlaway, K. (2014) *Promoting Health Behaviour: A Practical Guide.* 2nd edn. London: Routledge.

USA GOV: https://www.usa.gov

Vallone, D. M., Duke, J. C., Cullen, J., McCausland, K. L. and Allen, J. A. (2011) Evaluation of EX: a national mass media smoking cessation campaign. *Journal of Public Health,* 101 (2), 302–9.

Van de Sijpt, E. (2014) Complexities and contingencies conceptualised: towards a model of reproductive navigation. *Sociology of Health and Illness,* 36 (2), 278–90.

Varela, A. and Pritchard, M. E. (2014) Peer influence: use of alcohol, tobacco, and prescription medications. *Journal of American College Health,* 59 (8), 751–8.

Veenstra, G. and Burnett, J. P. (2014) A relational approach to health practices: towards transcending the agency-structure divide. *Sociology of Health and Illness*, 36 (2), 187–98.

Vygotsky, L. S. (1978) *Mind in Society. The Development of Higher Psychological Processes.* Cambridge, Massachusetts: Harvard University Press.

Wai Sze Lo, S., Ying Chair, S. and Kam Lee, F. (2015) Factors associated with health-promoting behaviour of people with or at risk of metabolic syndrome: based on the health belief model. *Applied Nursing Research*, 28, 197–201.

Wakefield, M. A., Loken, B. and Hornik, R. C. (2010) Use of mass media campaigns to change health behaviour. *Lancet*, 376, 1261–71.

Watson, J., Cunningham-Burley, S., Watson, N. and Milburn, K. (1996) Lay theorizing about 'the Body and Implications for Health Promotion'. *Health Education Research*, 11, 161–72.

Webb, O. J., Eves, F. F. and Kerr, J. (2011) A statistical summary of mall-based stair-climbing interventions. *Journal of Physical Activity and Health*, 8 (4), 558–65.

Webb, T. L., Joseph, J., Yardley, L. and Michie, S. (2010) Using the Internet to promote health behaviour change: a systematic review and meta-analysis of the impact of theoretical basis, use of behaviour change techniques, and mode of delivery on efficacy. *Journal of Medical Internet Research*, 12 (1), e4. Available at http://www.ncbi.nlm.nih.gov/pubmed/20164043

Weinreich, N. (2006) *What is Social Marketing?* Weinreich Communications. www.social-marketing.com

Weinstein, N. N., Marcus, S. E. and Moser, R. P. (2005) Smokers' unrealistic optimism about their risk. *Tobacco Control*, 14, 55–9.

Weintraub, D., Maliski, S. L., Fink, A., Choe, S. and Litwen, M. S. (2004) Sustainability of prostate cancer education materials: applying a standardized assessment tool to current available materials. *Patient Education and Counselling*, 55 (2), 275–80.

Wellings, K. and Macdowall, W. (2000) Evaluating mass media approaches to health promotion: a review of methods. *Health Education*, 100 (1), 23–32.

White, D. S. and Le Cornu, A. (2011) *Visitors and Residents: A New Typology for Online Engagement. First Monday*, 16 (9). Available at http://www.uic.edu/htbin/cgiwrap/bin/ojs/index.php/fm/article/viewArticle/3171/3049#author

Whiting, A. and Williams, D. (2013) Why people use social media: a uses and gratifications approach. *Qualitative Market Research: An International Journal*, 16 (4), 362–9.

Wiggins, S. (2008) Representations and constructions of body weight and body management. In Riley, S., Burns, M., Frith, H., Wiggins, S. and Markula, P. (eds) *Critical Bodies: Representations, Identities and Practices of Weight and Body Management.* Basingstoke: Palgrave Macmillan, pp. 23–6.

Wilkinson, I. (2001) *Anxiety in a Risk Society.* London: Routledge.

Wilkinson, I. (2006) Psychology and risk. In Mythen, G. and Walklate, S.

(eds) *Beyond the Risk Society: Critical Reflections on Risk and Human Society.* Maidenhead: Open University Press, pp. 25–42.

Wilkinson, T. M. (2013) Nudging and manipulation. *Political Studies*, 61, 341–55.

Williamson, L. (2014) Patient and citizen participation in health: the need for improved ethical support. *The American Journal of Bioethics*, 14 (6), 4–16.

Willig, C. (2000) A discourse-dynamic approach to the study of subjectivity in health psychology. *Theory and Psychology*, 10, 547–70.

Willig, C. (2008) A phenomenological investigation of the experience of taking part in 'extreme sports'. *Journal of Health Psychology*, 13, 690–702.

Windahl, S., Signitzer, B. and Olson, J. (2009) *Using Communication Theory: An Introduction to Planned Communication.* 2nd edn. London: Sage.

Winter, R., Fraser, S., Booker, N. and Treloar, C. (2013) Authenticity and diversity: enhancing Australian hepatitis C prevention messages. *Contemporary Drug Problems*, 40 (4), 505–29.

Woodall, J., Cross, R. and Warwick-Booth, L. (2012) Has empowerment lost its power? *Health Education Research*, 27 (4), 742–5.

World Health Organization (1998) *Health Promotion Evaluation: Recommendations to Policymakers Report of the WHO European Working Group on Health Promotion Evaluation.* Copenhagen: WHO Regional Office for Europe.

World Health Organization (1986) *Ottawa Charter for Health Promotion.* First International Conference on health promotion, 17–21 November, Ottawa, Copenhagen: WHO Regional Office for Europe.

World Health Organization 7th Global Conference (2009) Available at http://www.who.int/healthpromotion/conferences/7gchp/track2/en/

World Health Organization Commission on the Social Determinants of Health (2007) *Achieving Health Equity: From Root Causes to Fair Outcomes.* Geneva: World Health Organization. Available at http:// www.who.int/ social_determinants/resources/interim_statement/en/index.html

Wormeli, R. (2015) The 7 habits of highly affective teachers. *Educational Leadership*, 73 (2), 10–15.

Wright, N., Bleakley, A., Butt., Chadwick, O., Mahmood, K., Patel, K. and Salhi, A. (2011) Peer health promotion in prisons: a systematic review. *International Journal of Prisoner Health*, 7, 37–51.

Xiao, H. et al. (2014) Protection motivation theory in predicting intention to engage in protective behaviors against *schistosomiasis* among middle school students in rural China. *PLOS: Neglected Tropical Diseases*, 8 (10), e3246, doi: 10.1371/journal.pntd.0003246.

Yeo, M. (1993) Toward an ethic of empowerment for health promotion. *Health Promotion International*, 8 (3), 225–35.

Yeun, E. J., Baek, S. and Kim, H. (2013) Health promotion behaviour in middle-aged Koreans: a cross sectional survey. *Nursing and Health Studies*, 15, 461–7.

Young, M. (2005) In *Focus Programme on Skills, Knowledge and Employability*. National qualifications frameworks: their feasibility for effective implementation in developing countries. Skills Working Paper No. 22. Geneva: International Labour Office.

Zarcadoolas, C., Pleasant, A. and Greer, D. S. (2005) Understanding health literacy: an expanded model. *Health Promotion International*, 20 (2), 195–203.

Zinn, J. O. (2005) The biographical approach: a better way to understand behaviour in health and illness. *Health, Risk and Society*, 7, 1–9.

Index

Page numbers in *italics* denote a figure

DATE DUE
